HOW AND WHY OF YOGA AND MEDITATION

Marvels of the Mind
Part III
(Economy Edition)

Dr. King

ISBN-13: 978-1503011755
ISBN-10: 1503011755

Table of contents

Also by Dr. King

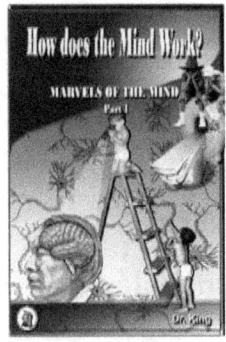 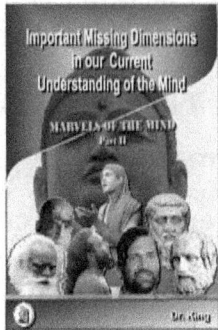 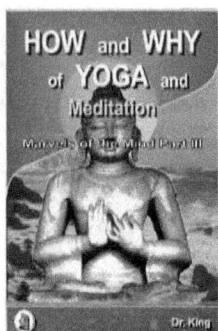

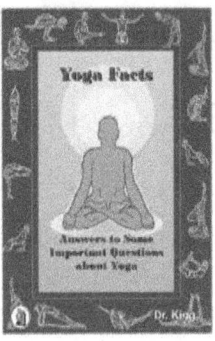 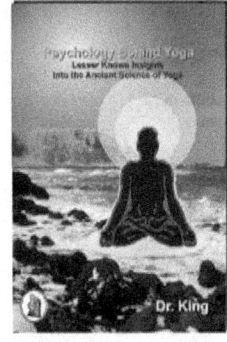 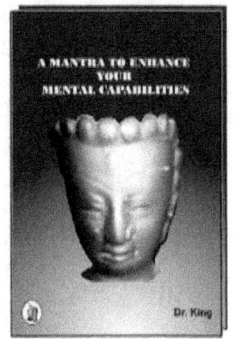

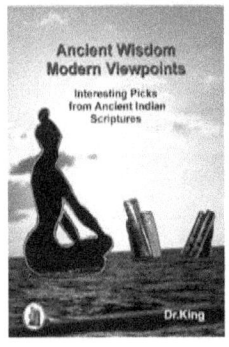 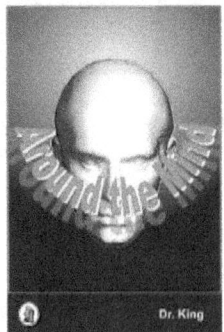

Prologue

Lot has been written about Yoga. However, predominant emphasis has been on Yoga postures and their health benefits. Most of the books on Yoga focus on "How" and "Why" aspects of performing various Yoga postures. There is no doubt that Yoga postures are beneficial in improving the health as indicated by several research reports.

But Yoga is not just body postures, as commonly believed. It has several other components that probably have a greater potential not only as health enhancers, but also as means to attain higher mental and spiritual levels.

The need of the hour is clarity on how Yoga achieves these results. Some scientific investigations have been conducted by various groups, but we are still not clear about the exact mechanism by which Yoga works. Better scientific understanding of the working of Yoga with all its associated processes is essential to reap complete benefit of this marvelous system.

The Yoga as proposed by Patanjali more than 2000 years ago is primarily about mind and its systematic modulation, to achieve various goals – from mundane stress reduction to ultimate realization.

The current book is meant to provide a clear understanding of various Yoga processes in the light of modern scientific knowledge. Most importantly, it tries to explain the "How" and "Why" of each of the Yoga processes in terms of neuroscience – the modern scientific effort to understand the mind. This gives better insight into the underlying mechanisms and clears lot of misconceptions.

The book is also a complete step by step guide detailing the "How" and "Why" of Yoga practice, for the benefit of those who would like to take it up seriously.

Overview of the book

In today's fast paced life style, the predominant problem seems to be stress. It is not surprising that almost two third of the health problems reported in the doctor's offices are either caused by stress or exacerbated by stress.

How does chronic stress cause health problems? This is the topic I discuss in Chapter 1. In that chapter, I also discuss the neural mechanisms that probably underlie stress.

Yoga attacks right at the root of stress. Two of the Yoga techniques that are often overlooked have great potential in minimizing stress. These two techniques are discussed in great detail in Chapter 2. This chapter also discusses how these techniques minimize most of the stress.

In Chapter 3, I discuss a non Yoga technique, albeit based on the ideas mentioned in Yoga, which is probably most beneficial for religiously oriented people with emotional bent of mind. Even Patanjali recommends this as a short cut to Yoga practice. Later in Chapter 6, I show how this technique can enable one to reach the same ultimate states that Yoga promises to take.

Most people mean Yoga postures when they talk about Yoga. Well known Yoga proponents and researchers are no exception. Yoga postures definitely have a great potential. But probably we are yet to understand it completely. in Chapter 4, I trace the historical roots of Yoga postures and discuss some scientific research into their efficacy. I also explain in a step by step manner, how some simple but very effective Yoga postures can be performed.

A healthy body with a stress free mind is definitely what most of us would like to have. But to make progress in life, this is not sufficient. We need to apply our mind in a focused manner to whatever we do in life. Yoga has simple techniques to sharpen our focusing skills. In Chapter 5, I discuss an assortment of Yoga as well as non Yoga techniques to improve our mental focus.

The crux of Yoga is meditation – a process during which all mental activities are shutoff step by step. I discuss this most important aspect of Yoga in Chapter 6. I give a step by step procedure explaining how one can go through various stages of meditation. I also explain "How" and "Why" of these stages, in scientific terms, providing lot of clarity into these poorly understood aspects of meditation.

What awaits on the other side of a completely calm mind? This is a question that transgresses the realms of reasoning, and even the boundaries of science! Reaching this 'state' is the real goal of Yoga. in Chapter 7, I try to explain this 'state' that is beyond the reach of explanation.

Not all people may be able to go through the entire set of processes enlisted in Yoga. But even practicing a subset of these processes can take one a long way. in Chapter 8, I suggest a small assortment of these processes that can be practiced by everyone. The benefits are more than worth the time spent on them. I hope that you will surely take advantage of.

Read on for an enlightening journey through Yoga.

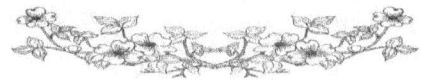

1 Stress is the prominent cause of problems

A survey conducted in the US reports that as high as 60% of Americans undergo great deal of stress at least once a week. Probably, similar figures apply to other developed nations as well. It is estimated that almost two-thirds of ailments reported in doctors' offices are either caused by stress or exacerbated as a result of stress. Stress can lead to diverse health problems: high blood pressure, diabetes, cardiac problems, obesity, arthritis, insomnia (sleeplessness), impotency, irregular menstrual cycles, early aging etc. to name only a few.

Several alternate therapies have been tried to alleviate adverse effects of stress, Yoga being one of the important ones. What is attractive about Yoga is that it is inexpensive and supposedly side effect free. Several research efforts report the efficacy of Yoga in not only managing stress related problems, but also in preventing stress from adversely affecting our health (see Chapter 4 for discussion on some research findings). Before we get into the details of how Yoga can help us, let us first look at how stress ultimately leads to health problems.

What is stress?

Almost all of us have experienced stress at some stage or other in our lives. But ironically it is difficult to clearly define what constitutes stress. Each individual experiences stress in a unique way and its perceived intensity varies from person to person. Scientists define stressor as any event that upsets the 'normal' functioning of our body (i.e. homeostasis).

In lower life forms, stress is almost always an external threat, from a predator for example. The victim has either to flee from the site of threat or to protect itself by fighting back: a flight or fight scenario. Our biological evolution has equipped us to handle this situation so that we can protect ourselves from external threats.

The stress we routinely go through is more psychological rather than physical. But surprisingly the basic mechanism adopted by the body to handle physical as well as the psychological stress is the same. The same systems get into action in both cases to prepare us to handle the stress.

How does the body react to occasional stress?

There are mainly three systems that come into play when we are faced with a stressor:
1. The voluntary nervous system.
2. The autonomous nervous system.
3. The neuro-endocrine system.

The role of these systems is primarily to make us ready to face the eventuality. Whether it is flight or fight, our brain has to send signals to our muscles to perform the needed act. More energy needs to be supplied to these muscles so that they can sustain their action. At the same time, the body needs to be kept fit and healthy, well protected from pathogens that may weaken it. All these would put the body in a high vigilant state. But once the threat subsides, our body has to be brought back to 'normal' state.

Let us briefly look at how each of these is achieved by these three systems that ready the body to handle the stress.

1. Voluntary nervous system: The voluntary nervous

system takes care of issuing appropriate signals to the muscles so that proper action can be taken. This is important in the case of external stress.

2. Autonomous nervous system: In order to enable

the muscles to act, they need to be supplied with more energy. The autonomous nervous system achieves this by pumping more blood to these muscles. The arteries connecting to these muscles are relaxed and the heart is made to pump more blood. Simultaneously, the blood flow to other areas of the body that are not involved in the flight or fight action is reduced. The body is hence put in a high state of alert to face the eventuality posed by the stressor.

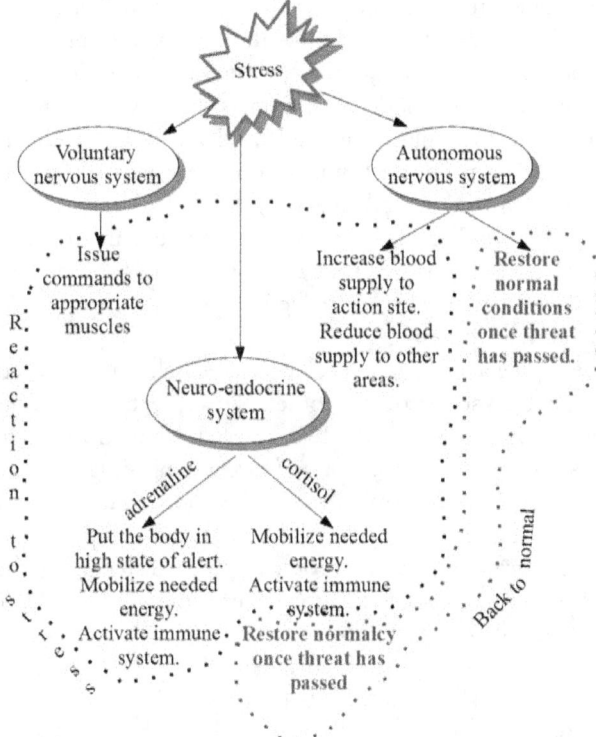

Figure 1.1 Body's response to occasional stress

This high state of alert can be damaging if kept for long. So, parts of the autonomous nervous system take care to bring the body back to the normal state once the stressor has passed. This action is very essential to prevent any damage.

3. Neuro endocrine system: This system produces various stress hormones that help the body in effectively handling the stress. The two major hormones are epinephrine (also known as adrenaline) and cortisol. These hormones in turn stimulate release of other hormones that have a series of effects. But, for the sake of brevity, I will keep referring to only these two hormones, though in reality several different hormones may be involved in the effect described.

Adrenaline puts the body in a high state of alert. It mobilizes energy and delivers it to muscles for the body's response.

Cortisol promotes energy replenishment. This it does by mobilizing energy into the bloodstream from storage sites in the body, by increasing cardiovascular tone, and by delaying long-term processes in the body that are not essential during a crisis, such as feeding, digestion, growth, and reproduction.

Cortisol and adrenaline facilitate the movement of immune cells from the bloodstream and storage organs such as the spleen into the tissue where they are needed to defend against infection. This fortifies our immune system.

Some of the actions of these hormones help to mediate the stress response, while some of the other, slower actions counteract the primary response to stress and help re-establish its normal balance.

Stress also enhances memory of threatening situations and events so that they can be remembered to take appropriate action in future recurrences of such events. The brain systems – dopaminogenic systems - that are involved in producing and distributing the neurotransmitter dopamine needed for several memory and other functions, get stimulated due to stress.

The overall strategy adopted by our body in response to occasional stress is as shown in Figure 1.1.

Normally, the body gets back to its normal state after the stress has passed. So, the response of the body for the stress helps the body in protecting itself. But that is not the case if the stress keeps recurring or remains for a prolonged duration of time, or in other words, it becomes chronic. Chronic stress can be harmful and can lead to several diseases as we will see in the next section.

What makes chronic stress harmful?

The response of the body to a stressor is meant to protect the body from the adverse effects of the stress. But ironically this very same response can damage the body when this stress gets prolonged over a period of time, or if it recurs time and again. This can lead to many diseases that I mentioned in the beginning of this chapter. How does this happen?

As can be seen from Figure 1.1 there is a pair of counteracting forces: one of them trying to put the body in a high state of alert and the other that tries to bring the body back to normalcy. In normal circumstances, i.e. when the stress is occasional or is for a short duration, these forces balance each other and no damage is done to the body and it passes off the stress with little adverse effect.

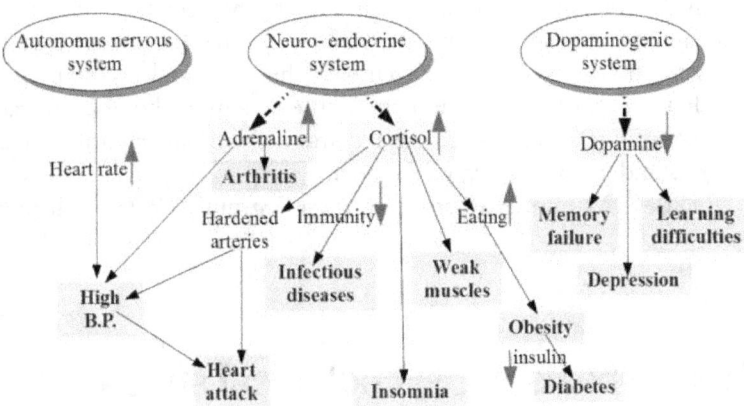

Figure 1.2 Some of the harmful effects of chronic stress

But when the stress becomes chronic, this balance gets disturbed: the mechanisms that put the body in high alert become more and more sensitive and the ones that counter them become more and more sluggish. This is to be expected since the body interprets continued stress as part of normal state of affairs and tries to remain vigilant all the time. But this is where the problem starts.

Over exposure to cortisol (due to chronic stress) can weaken muscles and it can result in hardening of arteries. This combined with increased heart rate can lead to high blood pressure and increased risk of heart attack. High levels of adrenaline also increase blood pressure.

High levels of cortisol affect the eating habits of the stressed individual. The eating becomes uncontrolled and results in obesity. Eating more than needed, results in fat stored in the body: obesity. Obesity is one of the prime causes of diabetes. Obesity with high cortisol level brings down insulin secretion over a period of time.

Sustained exposure to high levels of cortisol acts to suppress immune function. It also interferes with sleep onset resulting in lack of sleep. Sleep deprivation further raises cortisol levels, setting off a vicious cycle and finally leading to insomnia.

Stress for a short duration coaxes certain brain systems – dopaminogenic system - to produce dopamine so that the threatening event can be remembered and appropriate action be taken in future. But this very same mechanism goes awry when the stress becomes chronic. Prolonged stress adversely affects the secretion of neurotransmitters such as dopamine which are essential for learning, emotions and memory in general. Eventually this leads to depression.

High levels of adrenaline increase the activity of body chemicals that contribute to inflammation and these chemicals in turn lead to arthritis and possibly aging of the brain.

Figure 1.2 summarizes some of these harmful effects of chronic stress.

Neural basis of psychological stress

What we saw in the previous sections is how external stress is handled by the body and how chronic stress can be harmful. Most of the time the stress we come across in life are not physical but psychological: extreme competition for achievement, tight deadlines, threat to social acceptability, peer pressure, inability to keep up with time, uncertainty about future, a feeling of let down, a feeling of loss of control, and so on.

Each of these situations gives rise to mental events that may or may not have been directly triggered by the environment. Instead of a threat from an external attack, the threat is within - a conflict between opposing thoughts. If positive thoughts have an upper hand, we are safe. Otherwise, we are under stress.

Once we are under the clutches of negative thoughts and we do nothing to correct the situation, these thoughts generate more negative thoughts and their domination continues. Eventually we end up in chronic stress. Barring extreme pathological conditions, the generation of these thoughts has very much to do with the contents of our mind – prevailing mental setup, and inputs we acquire through our interactions with the environment.

Owing to evolutionary reasons, the way our body copes up with these psychological stresses is very similar to the way it handles externally driven stress threatening to cause physical harm. You probably have noticed some of these reactions – the heart beating rapidly, the breathing getting faster and so on – when you experience mental stress.

Before we see how thoughts can result in psychological stress, let us first see how thoughts are formed.

How are thoughts formed?

Our current scientific understanding has not yet reached a stage where we can completely explain the mechanisms behind the formation of thoughts. However, we do know that our brain continuously works even when we are not doing any sense perception or making any physical movements – i.e. when we not performing any task.

Using fMRI scanner, scientists have observed that certain regions of our brain get activated when we are not performing any task and this activity gets reduced when we are performing some task. Scientists suspect that these activities are due to thoughts that get generated in our mind. To be very specific, they call this activity as 'task unrelated thoughts' (TUT) to differentiate it from other class of thoughts that may be getting produced during the process of performing some task.

There are many types of task unrelated thoughts: thoughts about ourselves, thoughts about some problem that we are solving, thoughts pertaining to some imagination, and so on. The exact neural mechanisms underlying the formation of these thoughts are not yet clear. However, scientists suspect that the contents of various memories could be influencing the creation of these thoughts. For example, the autobiographical memories are believed to be responsible for the generation of thoughts about our emotions, our future planning, our goals and ambitions, our interactions with others, and so on – i.e. thoughts revolving around 'I'.

Let us look a bit more into the possible mechanisms of formation of thoughts. I presume the background provided in Part I of this book series for the discussion in this section, and also that in later chapters.

Thoughts as sporadically formed neural networks

As we saw in Part I of this book series, most neurons in our cerebral cortex are spare in the sense that they are neither part of any pre-connected specialized networks nor they are involved in memory storage, nor they play the role of messengers between different neural networks. Layers of these neurons are pre-connected in a random fashion but the synaptic strengths between them are not strong enough to perform any function. They become meaningful networks only when these connections become stronger.

In Part I, we saw how these connection strengths can vary depending on the activity that goes on in the vicinity of these neurons. Scientists observed that when slices of cortex from rat brains are artificially grown on a grid of electrodes, these neurons gradually develop stronger connections between them. Under favorable conditions, this activity can even burst out into what they call 'neuronal avalanches' implying a multiplying effect in the activity between these neurons.

Now coming back to the spare neurons in our brain, these too are interconnected in some random fashion with week synaptic connections. These neurons are surrounded by other neurons in the vicinity that could be very active. This activity induces activity in these spare neurons and they tend to form clusters of strongly connected neurons.

These sporadically formed neural networks encode our thoughts. Unlike in the experiment conducted by the scientists using electrode grids, these newly formed networks are not random but their formation is guided by the contents of pre-existing memory store, sense inputs, pre-existing thoughts and so on. That means their content is decided by our past experiences, emotions, and existing condition of our mind. However, formation of these networks is governed by the following considerations.

- When they are in the process of forming, the activity within them has to be sustained either by the activity of other already formed networks, or by the boosting provided by the attention system.

- Their activity should not be dampened by other networks that may compete with them.

- The attention system can guide the formation of these networks by selectively choosing existing networks that can influence – either positively or negatively - the network being formed.

If all conditions are favorable, then the synaptic strengths between the neurons in these new networks become stronger and a longer lasting network that encodes a specific thought gets formed. Or else the activity in these yet to be formed networks gradually dies down.

Several such sporadically formed networks can get formed. They either compete among themselves or support each other, depending on the content encoded in them. Thus they form 'coalitions' of networks that support like-networks and suppress networks of opposite kind.

The activity in a newly formed network induces further generation of new networks of like content. This proliferation of networks can go on unless checked by networks that oppose them.

All these thought networks not only compete among themselves but also vie to draw the attention of the attention system. The attention system could get overloaded by constant switching between these networks. This probably is the neural mechanism underlying psychological stress. To summarize, the psychological stress is caused due to

- Flurry of uncontrolled thoughts.
- Competition between rivaling thought groups.
- Overloading of the attention system, due to rapid switching between rivaling groups of thoughts.

With this background in mind, in the next chapter let us see how Yoga can help us in minimizing this psychological stress.

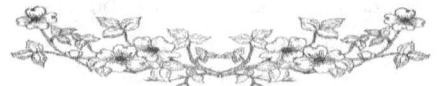

2 Yoga way to minimize stress

In the previous chapter we discussed how chronic stress can be harmful. We also saw how psychological stress is caused by conflicting thoughts, flurry of cascading thoughts, and the rapid switching of attention between these sporadically formed thoughts. We also briefly discussed the possible neural basis of these psychological stresses.

In this chapter let us move on to see how Yoga can help us in minimizing this stress. Though stress minimization is not the ultimate goal of Yoga, it is definitely a very useful byproduct. It is important to emphasize the point that Yoga may not be the remedy for acute pathological conditions that may need psychiatric intervention. However, use of Yoga as a supporting therapy in such cases may be worth considering. Yoga may also be useful as a prophylactic measure to prevent stress build up.

As we discussed in Chapter 1, the prominent cause of psychological stress is the conflict between negative thoughts and positive thoughts, and the overloading of the attention system. The thought conflict can be minimized either by minimizing the negative thoughts or by strengthening the positive thoughts so that ultimately the positive thoughts prevail. The load on the attention system can be minimized by restricting the thoughts to only the useful ones.

Accordingly, Yoga adopts a three pronged strategy to minimize stress. These three are as follows.

1. Block the source of negative thoughts.
2. Utilize positive reinforcement to boost positive thoughts.
3. Restrict the spurt of thoughts and channel them in a focused manner.

In this chapter, we will discuss the first two and postpone the third to later chapters. The first two form the first two steps, namely *Yama* and *Niyama* of Patanjali's eight-step Yoga (*Ashtānga Yoga*). We will see more on the eight steps in Chapter 6.

Most modern Yoga schools either ignore these two steps or give them cursory importance. As we can see in the following sections, full benefit of Yoga can be obtained only when we give a serious attention to these two important steps.

The source of negative thoughts

It may surprise many to know that the source of many of our negative thoughts lies in our present life style. Today we live in an 'individual centered' world. Suitability or otherwise of all our actions is judged merely based on how a given action is going to benefit 'me' or harm 'me'.

Anything that benefits 'me' is right and wrong otherwise. This is the root cause of conflicts and ensuing stress. We tend to forget that we cannot exist merely as individuals and our existence is closely tied to the existence of others around us. In our eagerness to do 'the right thing' - as judged by the 'individual centered' yard stick – we do harm to others and give rise to stressful conditions.

We need to look beyond just 'me'. Our actions should be guided by a macro view and not individual centered view. The set of do's and don'ts that are conducive to the well being of 'all' should be our guideline while we decide on suitability of any action. Ancient Indians called it *Dharma*.

Dharma is not any particular religion but the basis of all religions – whether eastern or western. Every religion emphasizes some aspects of this universal religion. The scope of 'all' in this *Dharma* may vary from religion to religion. In some, it may be restricted to members of a particular community, in some others, it may be restricted to human beings in general, and in more broader ones it embraces all living beings and may be non living beings as well. Patanjali is from this tradition that believed in universal *Dharma*.

Patanjali's Yoga lays emphasis on some of the key features of this *Dharma*. It may be impossible for us to stick to this *Dharma* to the core. But attempting to stick to it to the extent possible, can take us a long way.

Yama – the right way to stress free living

Yoga emphasizes mainly on five do's/don'ts. These are collectively called *Yama*. Patanjali's five do's/don'ts to block possible sources of stress are

1. *Ahimsa*
2. *Satya*
3. *Asthëya*
4. *Aparigraha*
5. *Brahmacarya*

Single word English translations of these, is difficult. Briefly put, these imply - don't hurt anyone, don't be dishonest, don't covet other's possessions, don't amass unnecessary wealth and don't indulge in uncontrolled sense pleasures. It is needless to say that a world free of fear, hatred, mutual distrust, greed, and over indulgence in sense pleasures is the most peaceful one.

Most religions emphasize these tenets in different ways and give varying importance to some of them. In religions like Buddhism, these form the core principles of the religion. Patanjali puts these down not as tenets of any religion, but as steps one has to abide by to prepare oneself for Yoga. Let us look at how Yoga defines them.

1. *Ahimsa*

In today's world of mutual hatred and resulting terrorism, Patanjali's first 'do' deserves prime importance. Patanjali calls it *ahimsa*. This word is generally translated as non violence. But what is violence? The definition of violence differs from person to person and from situation to situation.

Does attacking an enemy in a war field constitute violence? Does punishing a criminal for his crime amount to violence? Can repelling an aggressor to protect oneself and the fellow beings be termed as violence? Or slaughtering an animal in a 'humane' way enables it to be called non violent?

Actually, it is difficult to precisely define *ahimsa*. Probably it can be defined as 'not indulging in avoidable harm to someone'. Patanjali is well aware of the difficulty in defining *ahimsa* and says that it may differ from person to person, time to time, and from situation to situation. But he advocates *ahimsa* under all conditions. He promises a hatred free world when such *ahimsa* is practiced. Such a world will definitely be tension free and peaceful.

Many religions consider all living beings, excepting human beings, as creatures meant as food. So generally, most don't consider killing an animal for food as violence. But ancient Indians did not differentiate between humans and other beings when considering their right to exist. They felt that all should be given a fair chance to survive and thrive. But eating meat inevitably violates this tenet.

Does meat eating amount to violence? Most of us are non-vegetarians and at least in the affluent countries meat forms an important part of diet. Does slaughtering an animal constitute violence – even if it is done in a humane way? Ancient Indians always considered it so. It is not just how that animal suffers or does not suffer, but the fact that we are snatching its right to exist.

Interestingly, ancient Indians, unlike their modern upper caste counterparts, were almost always not strict vegetarians. Vedas do talk about animal slaughters conducted as part of various rituals.

But what is noteworthy is the fact that they still considered any kind of harm to fellow beings as unacceptable and they were apologetic about it. There are several passages in the Vedas where either a priest apologizes to the tree - the branches of which he had to cut for the use in a religious ritual, or prays on behalf of the animal - which he had slaughtered for the ritual, wishing its heavenly journey.

In all these cases, there is a hidden reminder that such violence should be avoided. Also, there is a justification given to such violence since the rituals were aimed at the greater benefit of all and violence to some was unavoidable in achieving that goal.

The ancient law-maker Manu, while giving out a long list of animals a person can consume, advocates non-violence! He justifies eating meat only when such meat is a left over from some religious ritual (*Yajnya Sësha*). Or in other words, only the meat offered to God can be consumed.

The remnants of this sentiment can be found in other religions as well. Whether it is ancient Judaism, or Islam, meat eating is allowed only when it is part of an offering to God. In all these cases there is a suggestion to avoid meat eating and the resultant violence to animals. The major emphasis on non-violence probably came from two of the religions that arose in ancient India, namely Buddhism and Jainism. Both these forbid violence. But strangely, some sects of Buddhism allow consumption of meat, while they still give lot of importance to non-violence.

Apparently, someone once asked the renowned Tibetan Buddhist monk Dalai Lama, whether he is a vegetarian. The great spiritual leader is supposed to have replied in the negative while stressing the point that he is trying to be one. In other words, there was always a stress on non-violence.

Another reason to be a vegetarian There is another reason for laying restrictions on meat consumption. Manu as well as other ancient Indian law-makers forbid meat eating also for the fact that it potentially affects mental makeup of a person.

Meat eating is supposed to enhance *rājasik* nature of a person as against *sātvik* one. A *rājasik* person is supposed to be action oriented and pleasure seeker as compared to a *sātvik* person who is supposed to be an intellectual and peace loving. As per this, too much meat consumption would make a person restless and pleasure hungry.

We do know from modern psychopharmacology that many of our mental disorders – hyperactivity, mania, bipolar syndrome, depression, and so on are due to abnormal production of neurotransmitters: either excitatory or inhibitory. In this context it will be interesting to explore the possibility - whether the food we consume, such as meat, has direct effect on the production of these neurotransmitters.

For the above cited reasons, some Yoga teachers emphasize on vegetarian diet for a Yoga practitioner. And some, knowing its impracticality, relax this restriction in a country specific manner!

If one takes the word nonviolence to the extreme, even eating any kind of food – vegetarian including – can be considered to be violence since even plants have life. That is the reason I defined non violence as 'non indulgence in avoidable harm to others'.

All along, we talked about violence in physical terms. But Patanjali takes the word violence to the extreme by saying that it is not just limited to physical harm but also to mental stress caused to another being, which constitutes violence. When a person acts dishonestly with a fellow being or even talks to him in a harsh way, it constitutes violence as per Patanjali. Avoidance of such dishonesty is crucial in minimizing stress. Patanjali calls it *Satya*.

2. *Satya*

In normal parlance the word *Satya* means truthfulness. The way the commentator of Yoga Sutra defines it, it is more about honesty rather than making a fact full statement. The literal meanings of sentences don't matter much but the intention behind them does. The way *Satya* is defined is as follows (as per the comments of the commentator Vyäsa on Yoga Sutra 1.30)

> *Satya is about being consistent between words and thoughts.*

> *One should convey only that which he has seen, heard and inferred, and only that which he has in his mind. In other words there should not be conflict between his words and thoughts.*

> *The purpose of communication is to convey right information. So it should be free from deceit. It should not be misleading nor should it be meaningless. It should not provoke violence.*

> *One should always speak the truth that is in the interest of all.*

In this context, the words of ancient law maker Manu (Manu Smrti

4.138) make lot of sense. He says

> *One should always speak the truth. One should*
> *say it in such a way that it does not hurt anyone.*
> *One should avoid telling harsh truths. So also un-*
> *truth even if it pleases someone. This is the ancient*
> *Dharma.*

Being dishonest has multiple problems – one is always afraid of being caught, one is busy finding excuses to cover up his dishonesty, one is in the danger of losing credibility and spoiling relations. So, it is always better to be honest. There may be temporary setbacks but it helps in the long run.

3. Asthëya

The Yoga Sutra commentator defines *Sthëya* (literally means theft) as acquiring things in violation of *Dharma*. Not indulging in *Sthëya* is *Asthëya*. What it means is that one should not acquire things that don't belong to him, or acquiring which has adverse effect on others. Even coveting someone else's possessions is wrong and a source of conflict.

4. Aparigraha

Amassing more than needed wealth is also a source of problems. In doing so, one not only has to spend his energy in the means to acquire it, but also worry about protecting it from others. Since amassing more than needed wealth almost always involves snatching someone else's share in the wealth, one may have to indulge in violence due to conflict of interest. Last but not the least; one tends to get preoccupied with the thoughts about how to spend that wealth. So, one should refrain from amassing more than needed wealth. This is called *Aparigraha*.

It is not always easy to decide what is essential and what is not. In a remote countryside with inadequate public transport, possessing a personal vehicle may be essential, whereas in a well connected city with good transport system; a personal vehicle may be a luxury. Similarly, eating enough to survive and be active cannot be considered overindulgence, whereas eating just to satiate the taste buds is. So, proper judgment needs to be used based on the circumstances and most importantly, governed by the rules of *Dharma*.

5. *Brahmacarya*

Patanjali's this 5th do in the list of *Yama* is often a source of debate. This word is used in different senses in different places in ancient Indian scriptures. It literally means 'the way a student lives with his teacher'. Patanjali does not clearly say what he means by this word. The commentator however defines it as 'control over sexual organs'. Probably he means 'control over sexual desires'. Many people who are desirous to practice Yoga get deterred by this definition since they find it impossible to abide by that.

However, considering the fact that Patanjali's Yoga is not about conserving sexual energy – unlike other later forms of Yoga – the commentator's words need not be taken literally. It could mean 'moderation in desires – sexual desire being one of them'. In this context, words of Manu (Manu Smrti 2.88, 2.94 and 2.2.96) with regard to how a student should be when he lives with his teacher (in residential schools) – the source of the word *Brahmacarya* - may make lot of sense.

The mind always gets distracted towards sense pleasures. But a student should rein in the senses the way an adept horse rider controls his unruly horse.

The senses can never be satiated completely by sense pleasures. More you indulge in sense pleasures; the more the desires get accentuated, like the fire that erupts when fuel is poured into it.

*It is impossible to completely control the senses or
totally abstain from sense pleasures, but one has to
ponder over the harm they cause and act in moderation.*

From these statements, it is clear that what is implied by the word
Brahmacarya is not complete abstinence but moderation, moderation
in all desires.

The above 5 do's/don't s minimize negative thought production. A
thought conflict can also be minimized by fortifying positive thoughts so that they can overpower the negative ones and eventually nullify
them. This is what Patanjali proposes in his next step of Yoga namely
Niyama. *Niyama* is a set of 5 do's that can potentially cultivate a positive outlook and minimize the effects of negativity.

Niyama –the way to reinforce positive thoughts

The five do's put down by Patanjali to reinforce the positive thoughts
are
1. *Sauca*
2. *Santosha*
3. *Tapah*
4. *Svädhyäya*
5. *Iswara pranidäna*

Again, it is difficult to provide single word English translations of
these Sanskrit words. Briefly put, these mean - maintain the body and
the mind clean, be content with what you have, be tolerant of vagaries of life, read right literature, and have faith in God. It is needless
to say that a mental makeup developed by these steps will be well
balanced and tranquil. Let us see these 5 do's one by one.

1. *Sauca*

Patanjali considers ill health as one of the causes of mental unrest (*vikshepa*) that eventually deter progress in Yoga practice. *Sauca* basically emphasizes the importance of keeping the body clean, consuming healthy food; and most importantly, keeping a clean mind filled with positive thoughts.

The commentator further adds that when one tries to keep the body clean, one becomes aware of the fact that the body is basically unclean and prone to defilement. This awareness, he says, would gradually free him from over association with the body as well as intimacy with others. This has shades of similarity with Buddhist meditative practices.

The Buddhists meditation practices suggest meditating on all kinds of 'dirty' objects – including a rotten corpse – just to come out of the attachment one has with his body. They call it right way of looking at things (*Vipassana*). These are techniques meant to use negative thoughts to achieve positive effects. For example, over attachment to body can be overcome by thinking about how filthy it is inside, and so on. Yoga does not use these techniques much, and I will skip further elaboration on them.

We can restrict the meaning of *Sauca* to mental and physical hygiene.

2. *Santosha*

Many of our mental worries are due to our dissatisfaction with what we already have – we are not as handsome or beautiful as the other person, we are not as rich or intelligent as someone else, and so on. Yoga teaches us to be content with what we have. This is what *Santosha* is all about.

This does not mean that one should not attempt to achieve higher levels of progress or perfection in life. Attempting to achieve perfection or progress is one thing, brooding over our inability to succeed in our attempts is yet another thing. As long as we try our best in a detached manner, it causes no harm.

3. Tapah

In spite our best efforts, we come across lot of hardships in life that are unavoidable. Instead of worrying over them, the right attitude is to bear with them to the extent possible. The vagaries in life should not perturb us and we should take them with a calm mind. This is *Tapah*.

4. Svädhyäya

Our mental makeup often depends on what we read, what we hear and what we discuss with others. If we read crime thrillers or erotic novels all the time, it is hard to keep a calm mind. In doing so we are unnecessarily perturbing our mind. Instead, we should read/ ponder over things that generate positive thoughts.

Most religious literatures provide you such a frame of mind. If you are a Christian, you may get solace by reading Bible; if you are a Muslim, you may find it in reading Quran; or if you are a Hindu, Bhagavad Gïta may infuse the same positive mental makeup. So, depending on one's background, one should read right literature. This is *Svädhyäya*.

5. Ïswara pranidäna

Life is full of unpredictable events that are beyond our control. To some extent we can develop immunity to such events by practicing *Tapah* as discussed earlier. But not all can do it. For such people, faith in God- or *Ïswara* as Patanjali refers to him - gives a ray of hope and a relief from the torments of life. This hope ensues from the belief that some super power such as God would eventually take us out of that problem. That is a strong positive thought that has the potential to nullify many negative thoughts.

Interestingly, the companion school of Yoga namely the Sänkhya almost denies the existence of God (refer to Part II of this book series). But Patanjali suggests faith in God as a way of making progress in Yoga. How does Patanjali define this God? Patanjali defines (Yoga

Sutra 2.24, 2.25, 2.26) God as follows.

> *Íswara is a special soul who is not affected by any*
> *worldly torments; one who is beyond any limits; one*
> *who is omniscient; one who is beyond time and the*
> *one who is the Guru of all Gurus.*

This is a very broad definition of God matching with the definition of God in most theistic religions. Patanjali says that surrender to this God can take us further in Yoga practice and enables us to attain the ultimate goal of Yoga. This is so because, the God is merciful and he is capable of removing all hindrances to the practice.

How does one go about praying to this God? Patanjali's suggestion is to meditate on 'Om' the symbol representing this God. We will see more on meditation later on.

For all those who are religiously oriented and predominantly emotional, there is a simpler way. Surprisingly, this simple way not only gives us peace of mind but also can potentially take us to the zenith of Yoga even without practicing Yoga! We will see this alternative to Yoga in the next chapter.

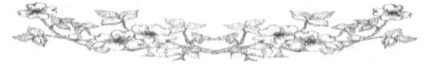

3 Sing your stress away

What I am going to discuss in this chapter is not part of Yoga. I am only building on the *Īswara pranidāna* talked about by Patanjali as a way to minimize stress and to make progress in Yoga. I call it devotional singing. As I show later on (in Chapter 6), devotional singing can even be an independent path to reach the same goals as that of Yoga. It is more suitable for emotionally oriented people with strong religious faith.

Almost all religions have a way of devotional singing. A Christian may call it carol; a Hindu may call it *Bhajan* or *Kirtan*. There is an opinion that Islam forbids singing. But I am sure it does not bar devotional singing. There is a class of Muslim saints called *Sufis*, who are well known for devotional singing.

There are two main aspects to devotional singing – the faith aspect where the devotee believes that God listens to his singing and relieves him of his agony. The other one – more analytically oriented one – sees devotional singing as one easy way of modulating the mental processes.

I would not like to go much into the former, since it is faith based and quite subjective in nature, precluding any analysis. In the latter, the existence or otherwise of God is immaterial. I am not implying that faith is unfounded, but an analytically explainable aspect fits more in the framework of things I discuss in this book.

To be effective as a stress reliever, the devotional singing has to meet certain criteria and should be done in a specific way. Let us first see the criteria for right way of singing.

Some do s and don't s about devotional singing

Devotional singing definitely involves singing. But it is not a musical concert. The purpose of the former is either religious or imparting peace to mind; whereas the purpose of the latter is mainly entertainment. Music definitely helps in focusing the mind, soothing the mind, and as a general motivator. But over emphasis on music can defeat the purpose.

The music employed in devotional singing has to be melodious, rhythmic with gradual changes in sounds. It should avoid harsh notes and shouting that are typical of some of the modern forms of music. For this reason, it is preferable to use classical music for devotional singing.

Any kind of pomp or show associated with devotional singing is also not advisable. That will have adverse effect on the mental processes. Basically that leads to craving for public attention. Craving leads to ego if sufficient attention is received and depression if no such attention is received. Though most people would like to sing in chorus, singing alone in a quiet place is more effective, with or without accompanying instruments.

Avoid negative thoughts

Devotional singing is generally some sort of conversation with God. But one should take care not to include concepts that depress the mind or provoke it to passions or craving. All negative thoughts should be avoided.

If you are a Christian, it is better to focus more on love, compassion, tolerance and such other divine qualities of Jesus Christ and not on the suffering he went through in the hands of his adversaries, or his agonizing crucifixion.

Similarly, if you are a Muslim, concentrate more on the mercy, kindness of almighty Allah, his promise to take care of all his devotees and so on, and not on the blood shedding that the Prophet and his followers had to suffer in the early days of Islam. A Hindu should avoid songs revolving around erotism – such as those describing purported erotic pastimes of say Krishna, songs focusing on self condemnation, or songs involving fierce depiction of Kali or some such God.

Devotional songs should not be a list of demands for favors. Devotion is an expression of undemanding love towards God. As far as possible, the songs should not ask for anything from God other than his love and kindness. Making a demand for any kind of material comforts or objects would only incite craving for them and ultimately dissatisfaction or disillusion. So it is better to avoid them.

Is devotional singing inferior to Yoga?

Some people entertain a false notion that devotional singing is for less intellectual people. It is true that devotional singing needs faith in God and does not involve much intellectual activity. But, as I will show in the next section and later in this book, devotional singing can also take one through various stages that Yoga promises to take. There were great Yoga practitioners like Ramakrishna Paramahamsa (Guru of Swami Vivekananda) who could easily go into *Samadhi* – the ultimate state of Yoga - just by devotional singing.

In India, devotional singing is treated on par with practice of Yoga, or the heights reached through intellectual pursuits (*Jñāna Yoga*). In fact, the author of *Nārada Bhakti Sutra* (a treatise on devotion) considers devotion to be superior to all other forms of spiritual practices including Yoga, ritualism, or *Jñāna Yoga*.

So one should not harbor such wrong notions about devotional singing, but take advantage of this simple and effective method especially if you are religious. It is an easy and natural way to peace.

How should one sing?

There are mainly two ways of devotional singing. The first one – the most common one – is to sing with a personified God as the focus.

The other one involves singing about an abstract notion of God.

In this section, I will touch upon both these forms of devotional singing. Neither of these is better than the other. Depending on your mental makeup and religious background, you can choose either or both.

Devotion to God as a person

Most religions view God as a person. This person may or may not have a form, but he is generally attributed with several human like emotions – love, mercy, anger and so on. The one to one relation one has with this person is called devotion. In most religions, this relation is like the relation between the master and his subordinate. The master is the protector, the provider; and the subordinate is the one who takes refuge in his master.

In general, this relation between God and devotee can be more than just the relation between master and subordinate. A Hindu sees it in many ways. It could be a relation between

▶ master and his slave – God being the master and the devotee his slave

▶ parent and a child – God being the mother or father and the devotee being the child

▶ child and mother - God is the child and the devotee is the mother!

▶ two friends – equality relation

▶ two lovers – God being the male and the devotee being the female

Traditional Indian devotional singing has songs depicting each of these forms of love to God, including even erotic songs depicting purported love between Krishna and his female companions. However, it is better to avoid the latter since they can negatively divert the mind.

Let me give some examples of various forms of devotions that are commonly found in Indian devotional singing. I have specifically taken Indian examples since one can find a rich variety of devotional songs and India has a long tradition of devotional singers. It also has elaborate treatises written specifically on devotion as a means to spiritual practice.

The examples I have used here for illustration are taken from different Indian languages and I am only providing simple English translations of some snippets to drive home the concept.

One devotee sings

"Oh God! They say that you are formless, devoid of any emotions. But I don't believe that. For me you are my master and I am your slave..."

Another one with some knowledge about the Vedas says

"The Vedas declare that you are formless. But no, I don't agree. I am sure that you are both formless and with form. Even if you are formless, please for my sake, assume some form and come to me because I cannot perceive something that has no form..."

Another devotee takes solace in the belief that his master always takes care of him. He sings

"The way he waters even the trees on top of a hill, the way he provides food to each and every bird or insect in a forest, the way he feeds even a frog that can survive inside a crevice in a rock, in the same way that very same God also takes care of me. So why should I grieve? Oh mind don't be perturbed, have patience..."

A devotee who views the God as a child sings

"Place your delicate feet on my heart and descend down. Please open your eyes and look at me for a

second, I am waiting for you with whatever I have to offer...

"You are so beautiful and there is none more beautiful than you. It is a pleasure seeing your divine form. I feel like gazing your tender rosy cheeks again and again...

"Don't cry my child. When I come back from my work I will bring you anklets. One of these days I will even bring you a beautiful dress. So, don't cry my dearest one...

"My dear child, you normally sleep on the galactic ocean and you are like the vast blue skies. You are the one who bestows extreme bliss to me. Let me rock your cradle and sing you a lullaby. Please go to sleep, please sleep...

On the other hand, the devotee who sees God as his real mother sings

"When I was in my mother's womb, you are the one who nourished me. And when I came out to this world, you are the one who produced milk in my mother's breast so that I could feed on that. I know that you are the one who always takes care of me. I never have to worry about anything...

"Oh Mother, the most beautiful, I am content with whatever you have given me. If at all, give me more devotion to you...

*"Of course, I make mistakes. At times, I get lured
by various sense pleasures and. I forget you completely. Please forgive me since I am your child and
as a mother you have to overlook your child's fol-
lies...*

Yet another devotee even expresses romantic feelings towards God
whom he considers as his lover

*"My Lord! My eyes are thirsty to see you; I do not
want to see anything but you. Your thoughts make
me forget everything. I am unable to concentrate on
my daily chores and I end up doing all kinds of sil-
ly things. Please come to me...*

*"When my eyes are filled with your charming form,
how can they crave for anything else? Nothing in
this world lures me. They (i.e. worldly things) are
like a traveler who goes away when he sees a guest
house that is already full...*

In another song the lover devotee says

*"I am seeing you inside me as well as outside. I am
seeing you everywhere. Even while dreaming I
dream only about you. Oh God! Am I going
mad!..*

Sometimes a devotee, who considers God as his friend, even engages
in mock fights

*"Oh God! Why are you so cruel? You have no
mercy on me at all. I have heard that you always
take care of your devotees. But why are you ignor-*

ing me? Did those other devotees bribe you or were
they your close relatives?..

"There is none in this world who is really benefited
by trusting you. Even a beggar would get nothing if
he solicits alms in your name...

"If you really consider yourself to be merciful, then
come at once and take me in your arms...

Devotion to God as an abstract concept

A Hindu not only treats God as master, friend, mother, child, lover
and so on; but also as an abstract all pervading concept. Accordingly,
typical Indian devotional songs could be quite abstract. Let me give
some examples.

"Oh God! The leaves sway when you breathe; the
flowers bloom when you smile. You are the one who
does everything and also the one who makes every-
thing happen. I surrender to you...

"You are the one who resides in a poor man as
well as in an enlightened person. Whatever I eat,
whatever I see around, whatever I feel and sense are
all your forms. There is nothing that is not you...

As you can see, in all examples I have given above, the meaning
of the words is also important and not just the rhyme or music. This
is important as I explain below.

Lyrics of a song evoke emotions

Emotions are essential in devotional singing. And it is the lyrics of a song that evoke appropriate emotions. The music may provide the motivation for singing, but it is the meaning of the song that really makes the difference, at least in the initial stages.

While singing, one should not only understand every word of the song, but also visualize, feel and experience it. The emotions expressed by the song should be felt while singing. This experience should be reflected in the voice modulation, facial expression and other body language. In intensely emotional songs, tears should automatically flow down from the eyes as if whatever is expressed in the song is real. In other words, the singer should get fully involved in the scenario created by the song, completely forgetting whatever that is happening around him.

Such total involvement may look quite impossible. But there are umpteen number of great devotees who could easily get into such moods. Ramakrishna Paramahamsa that I mentioned earlier is just one of them.

How does devotional singing work?

You probably wonder how such emotionally charged singing can really help in minimizing stress! First of all, while listing the don't s I have intentionally excluded certain emotions that can interfere in the process of stress elimination. The rest of the emotions though may look intense, can actually help in minimizing stress.

As I said earlier, I am restricting my discussion only around analyzable aspects of devotional singing. I am not implying that God does not exist and he has no role in whatever is happening. What I want to stress is that apart from religious faith, there are other aspects of religious singing that can make it useful as a means to stress reduction.

Let me digress a bit and take up an interesting approach a farmer friend of mine follows when he grows chilli peppers in his field. These pepper plants are prone to insect infestation and normal insecticide sprays are not very effective, besides being harmful to the consumers. My friend follows a simple harmless way. He grows rows of marigold plants interspersed with pepper plants. It seems, these insects love marigold plants more than the pepper plants and keep themselves busy feeding on them, sparing the pepper plants. By the time they finish off the marigold plants, peppers would be ready for harvesting, and no harm done to them!

I am giving this example to explain how devotional singing works especially if one is emotionally oriented. Emotionally oriented people suffer because of their intense emotions. They cannot express their emotions since that may end them in external conflicts or other entanglement. At the same time, suppressing the emotions often gives rise to mental stress. What devotional singing does is to provide an outlet to these emotions so that they do not affect mental peace. This is like the farmer in the above example diverting the insects to marigold plants!

There is yet another reason why devotional singing works. Most of the devotional songs express love to God. It is a scientifically proven fact that when someone is in love – romantic or otherwise, the brain suppresses all negative thoughts, while highlighting positive ones. This effectively reduces stress. Added to this, religious faith, expectation of well being, assurance of being taken care of etc. can also psychologically help the person.

There is a bonus which the devotional singer gets in addition. Properly done devotional singing can be very pleasurable, the pleasure often exceeding that derived from sense pleasures. But unlike the sense pleasures that have limitations, this divine pleasure is limitless. Even this aspect makes the depressed person forget his worries.

In the long run, continued practice of devotional singing can also take the mind to higher levels that Yoga can take. I will come to this aspect later on.

So far we saw how stress can be minimized either by practicing Yoga or by devotional singing. In Chapter 1 we saw how minimization of stress can help us in either preventing health problems or minimize the chances of illness getting worse.

Many people view various Yoga postures as health enhancers. In the next chapter we will look into this usage of Yoga as health enhancers.

4 Yoga postures as health enhancers

It is a common experience that when we are ill, our mind tends to be more irritable. Needless to say that physical health plays a very important role in deciding our mental well being. Even Patanjali cites illness as one of the hindrances to Yoga practice. Many of us take to Yoga mainly as a health enhancer.

Most people mean just the body postures when they talk about Yoga. Even adept Yoga teachers and practitioners are no exception in giving more than needed emphasis to this aspect of Yoga. In most scientific studies investigating the effectiveness of Yoga, body postures receive predominant attention. Is Yoga mainly a body oriented system? Are Yoga postures really beneficial in improving our physical health? What does the evidence say?

Before we answer these questions, let us see whether the Yoga postures that we know today have any historical support.

Historical support for Yoga postures

There are claims that evidence for Yoga postures can be found even in the ruins of 5000 year old Indus valley civilization (many of these ruins are found along present day India Pakistan border). But many of these evidences are not undisputed.

There are also people who believe that Yoga postures had always been in practice in ancient India from time immemorial. But recorded history is not so strong on evidence for postures being part of Yoga.

The ancient Buddhists who had elaborate Yoga like system emphasized more on meditative aspects. The ancient Buddhist texts namely the *Tipitakas* (~300 B.C.) talk about codes of conduct like *Yama* and *Niyama* of Yoga (called *vinaya*), breathing techniques similar to *Pränäyäma* of Yoga (called *änäpäna sati*), meditation techniques like *dhyäna* of Yoga (called *vipassana*) and even different stages of *samädhi* (up to 8 stages of *jhaanas*). But there does not seem to be much evidence for body postures that we find as part of Yoga today.

It may surprise many that the well known proponent of Yoga, namely Patanjali (~200 B.C.), makes no mention of the Yoga postures - as we know of them today - in his Yoga Sutra. He does mention about Yoga postures – which he calls *asana* – as the 3rd step of his eight step Yoga process. In Patanjali's words (Yoga Sutra, 2.46)

Asana is that which is stable and comfortable

Patanjali does not give any more details about asanas. From the definition it seems that he is referring to some postures that are useful during prolonged meditation. I will discuss why such postures are needed, which postures are suitable, and so on in Chapter 6.

The well known commentator of Yoga Sutra, namely Vyäsa (~500 A.D.) however lists some of the Yoga postures that are known today. The asanas that Vyäsa lists are *Padmäsana, Viräsana, Bhadräsana, Svastikäsana, Dandäsana, Paryankäsana, Krauncanishadanäsana, Hastinishadanäsana,* and *Ushtranishadanäsana.*

Among these, at least the first 4 are known to be postures useful for prolonged meditation. But Vyäsa does not describe how these asanas are performed. The only hint is in their names, for example, *Hastinishadanäsana* means the way an elephant (*Hasti*) sits.

A more detailed description of some these asanas can be found in much later text namely *Hatayoga Pradeepika* by Swami Svätmäräma (~ 15th century A.D.). This text lists around 15 asanas that include some of those listed above. Along with a brief description of how they are performed, this text also gives the benefits of performing them – health as well as spiritual.

Further texts dealing with variants of Yoga, belonging to later periods, add more and more asanas to Yoga practice. For example, *Shat-chakra Nirüpana* of Pürnänada (~ 16th century A.D.) and *Gherand Samhita* (author, period uncertain– probably 17th-18th century A.D.) mention about 32 asanas; while *Shivasamhita* (author, period uncertain – probably 17th-18th century A.D.) talks about 84 asanas but describes only 4.

It appears that originally the asanas were meant mainly as aides to keep the body stable and distraction free during long periods of meditation. Their role as physical health enhancers is something that seems to have developed over a long period of time.

Modern Yoga teachers however talk about hundreds of asanas. Almost all these teachers emphasize on their health benefits. More and more new asanas are added to this repertoire by modern Yoga teachers. The historical support for most of these asanas is uncertain. Nor their specific health benefits are consistently defined and scientifically verified. But still, the health benefits of asanas in general have been the focus of many research investigations.

Scientific evidence for Yoga postures as health enhancers

As I said earlier, the word Yoga is often used to mean Yoga postures. In sections that follow, I generally use it that way.

There are hundreds of research papers reporting various health benefits of Yoga. Many of these research efforts are either sponsored by institutions that propagate a specific form of Yoga or are conducted by Yoga teachers expounding a particular mode of practice. Some of these research efforts follow well defined procedures for investigating such alternative approaches to health care and their findings are published in reputed forums.

According to these studies, Yoga seems to be beneficial in almost every type of illness or at least can be used as a complimentary therapy. Most of these studies emphasize on beneficial effects of asanas. Before we arrive at any conclusions on these studies, let us see some of the prominent reported results.

How does Yoga help in improving health?

Yoga seems to correct the adverse effects of chronic stress that we discussed in Chapter 1. In terms of measureable parameters, a number of studies have shown that practice of Yoga decreases levels of salivary cortisol, blood glucose, as well as plasma rennin levels, and 24-hour urine norepinephrine and epinephrine levels.

Yoga is also believed to significantly decrease heart rate and systolic and diastolic blood pressure. Studies suggest that yoga reverses the negative impact of stress on the immune system by increasing levels of immunoglobulin as well as natural killer cells.

Yoga has been found to decrease markers of inflammation such as high sensitivity C-reactive protein as well as inflammatory cytokines such as interleukin-6 and lymphocyte-1B.

The exact mechanism how Yoga achieves these results, is not known. Nor we clearly know which aspect of Yoga actually brings in these effects. Scientists suspect that some aspects of Yoga 'somehow' enhance the soothing effects of neuro-endocrine and the autonomous nervous systems that we discussed in Chapter 1. These natural mechanisms built into the body to bring back the body to normalcy go haywire when one undergoes prolonged stress. And Yoga seems to put them back on track.

Yoga in the treatment of different health problems

Several scientific studies have shown that Yoga can be useful in managing several health problems. More importantly, Yoga has been found to be beneficial in treating arthritis, persistent pain especially chronic back pain, anxiety, and depression. You can find a small list of studies done to evaluate the effectiveness of Yoga in the **Bibliography**.

But the interesting point to note is that most of these studies mean Yoga postures when they talk about Yoga. If you see closely, even these Yoga postures involve several components namely

- Specially designed stretching exercise. This is the aspect that is often given the most emphasis.

- Delicate balancing of the body that requires complete mental concentration.

- Controlled breathing that is often synchronized with different stages of a Yoga posture
- Mental conditioning due to the wide spread publicity given to its health benefits

These components may make different contributions to the effect of a specific Yoga posture. Since most studies focus mainly on exercise part of Yoga postures, they compare health benefits of Yoga postures with that of routine physical exercises and try to show that they are markedly better than routine exercises. But the contributions of other components of Yoga postures are overlooked.

In these studies, often the word 'Yoga' is used to imply exercise part of Yoga postures, but in reality what is measured is the combined contribution of not only different components of Yoga postures, but also different Yoga processes themselves, as we will see in the next section.

Is 'Yoga' better than routine exercise?

The important question about Yoga postures is - do they have any added advantage as compared to physical exercises such as stretching, cycling, jogging, rigorous walk or aerobic exercises? This was the focus of one study conducted in 2010. This study investigated 12 different research efforts by different groups of researchers.

More than 800 subjects were part of these 12 research efforts. In each case, the benefit of 'Yoga' was compared to that of routine exercise. The 'Yoga' practiced by these subjects, generally involved not just postures, but meditation and controlled breathing (*Pränäyäma*) as well. That means it involved almost complete system of Yoga. The duration of the study was anywhere from 5 weeks to 24 weeks. Different groups used different criteria for evaluating the improvement using Yoga.

As many as 37 different parameters were used, ranging from precisely measurable body parameters such as blood glucose levels, to subjective criteria like quality of life.

It was found that Yoga excelled or was at least equal to routine exercise in most cases. In 22 out of 37 parameters Yoga was better, in

10 parameters Yoga and exercise both performed equally, and in the rest 5 parameters exercise was better than Yoga. The exercises that outperformed Yoga happened to be aerobic exercises and the parameters in those cases were supposed measure physical fitness.

Some observations

Though these results are definitely in support of Yoga, they are misleading in a way that the benefit of the entire system of Yoga is taken as that accrued by just Yoga exercise. As I said, Yoga is not just exercise. Not just the meditation and controlled breathing, even the asanas have components that calm the mind.

Complete mental concentration needed to stay in a given delicate body posture, the rhythmic breathing that is often clubbed with different stages of an asana have their own contributions to calming of the mind. As we saw in earlier chapters, calming of the mind is definitely a strong contributor to health enhancement. More research needs to be conducted to separate different aspects of Yoga postures, and understand the role and importance of each.

Having said this let me now give a small set of Yoga postures that are believed to be beneficial.

Some simple Yoga postures

The postures I describe in this section are relatively easy and safe to perform. But they provide exercise to the entire body and are believed to have several health benefits. Further, when these postures are done in a specific sequence, with associated breathing regime, they are supposed to bestow the benefits of controlled breathing (Pränäyäma) as well. I will talk about controlled breathing in Chapter 5.

Some of these postures have minor variants and are known by alternate names. Sometimes a single posture is divided into two postures. In this section however, I will focus mainly on one version of these postures.

Let me start with these postures one by one.

1. The Folded palms posture (*Namaskārāsana*)

Figure 4.1Folded palms posture (Image courtesy Dr. Omkar)

This is the simplest of all. Just stand erect, your feet laid flat on the ground and touching each other. Flex the elbows and join both the palms as shown in Figure 4.1..The thumbs (back edge) should be touching the chest. Breathe in and out calmly.

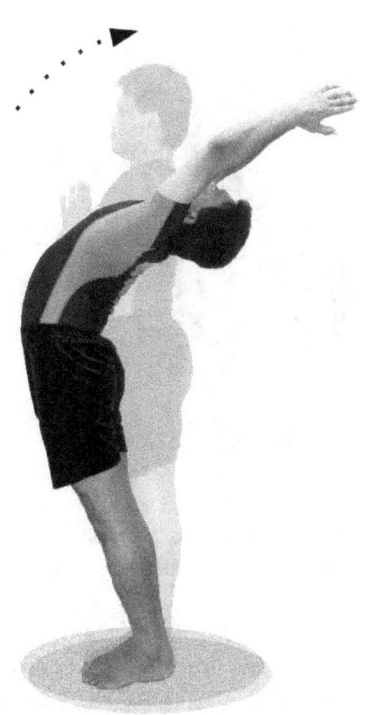

igure 4.2 Back ward bend posture (Image courtesy Dr. Omkar)

2. The Backward bend posture (*Urdhvāsana*)

Some schools call this posture as *Urdhvanamanāsana* . To do this, first stand in the *folded palms posture* described earlier. Slowly raise the folded palms up with arms stretched straight. Breathe in slowly while doing that. With slow inhalation, slowly bend backwards with the arms held as they are. Your gaze should be fixed towards the sky as if you are saluting the skies. The final posture is shown in Figure 4.2

Benefits: This posture is supposed to give good exercise to the spinal cord. It is also supposed to improve digestion, overcome constipation, and strengthen the waist.

3. The Forward bend posture (*Utthānasana*)

Start with the *backward bend posture* explained above. With slow exhalation slowly bend forward. Separate the folded palms and move the

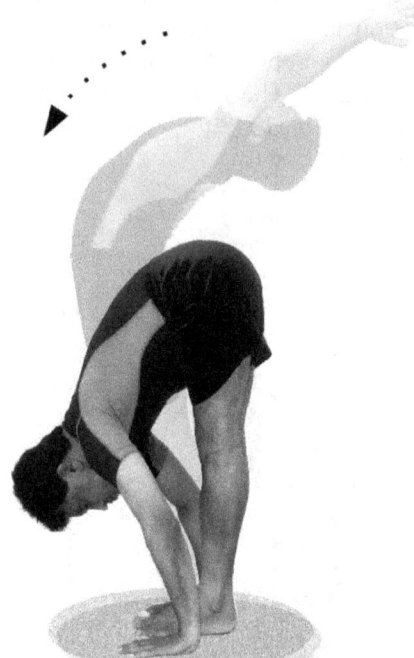

palms down so as to touch the ground one on either side of the feet as shown in Figure 4.3. As far as possible, ensure that the palms are held flat on the ground, and the knees don't buckle forward. It may be a bit difficult in the beginning, but practice should improve it. In any case, don't over strain yourself.

Some variants suggest touching the head to the knees. This posture is also called as *Hastapādāsana* by some.

Figure 4.3 Forward bend posture
(Image courtesy Dr. Omkar)

Benefits: This posture provides exercise to waist and it strengthens the thighs, knees and lower legs.

4. The One leg stretch posture (*Ekapāda prasaranāsana*)

Being in the *forward bend posture* explained above, slowly stretch one of the legs backward, while folding the knee of the other. Inhale slowly while doing this. The hands and the palms should be as they are. The back stretched leg should have its knee touching the ground as shown in Figure 4.4 . Fix your gaze forward.

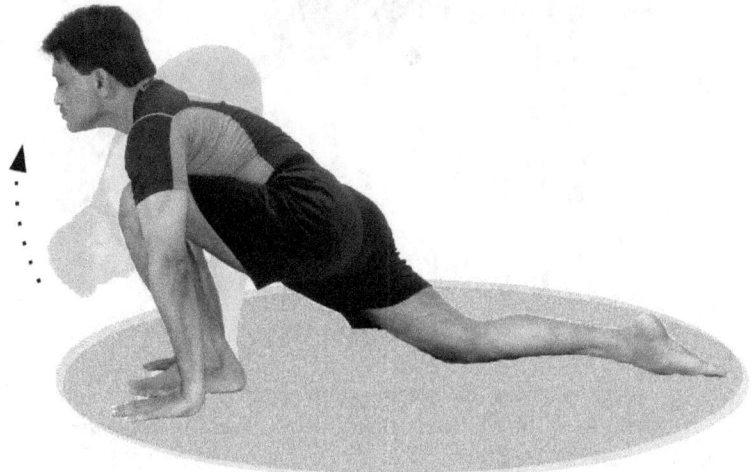

Figure 4.4 One leg stretch posture (Image courtesy Dr. Omkar)

Alternate the legs each time you perform this posture so that both legs get equal exercise.

Benefits: This posture is supposed to strengthen the muscles in the hips, thighs and lower legs. It is also supposed to relieve stiffness in the bottom portion of the spine.

5. The Both legs stretch posture (*Dvipādaprasaranāsana*)

Start with the *one leg stretch posture* described above, with one leg stretched and the other folded. While exhaling slowly, move the other leg also backward like the first one. Now lift the hips upwards so that the back remains parallel to the ground as shown in Figure 4.5.

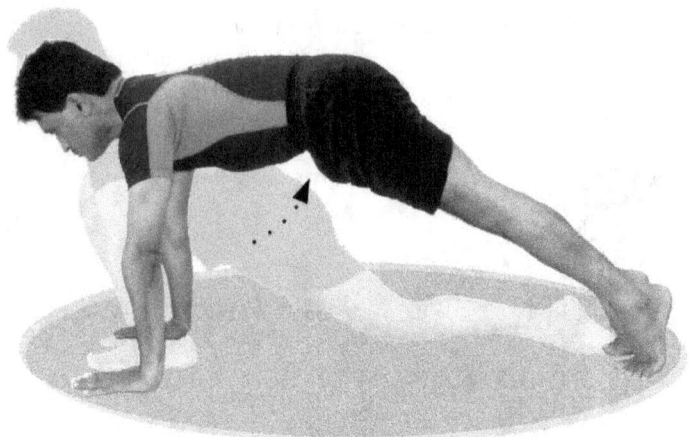

Figure 4.5 Both legs stretch posture (Image courtesy Dr. Omkar)

Some variants don't lift the hips, but keep the back in line with the stretched legs. The current posture is called the *mountain posture* (*Bhoodharāsana*) by some.

Benefits: This posture is supposed to strengthen calf muscles and relieve constipation.

6. The Stick posture (*Caduranga Dandāsana*)

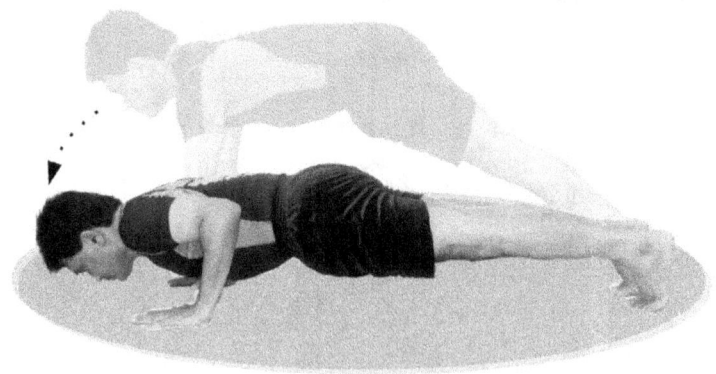

Figure 4.6 Stick posture (Image courtesy Dr. Omkar)

Starting from *both legs stretch posture* explained above, gradually lower the trunk while folding the elbows. The head, neck, trunk and the legs should be in a straight line and parallel to the ground. The entire body should be rested only on the palms and the toes as shown in Figure 4.6. No part of the body other than the palms and toes should touch the ground.

Benefits: This posture is supposed to strengthen the elbows and the shoulders since the weight of the entire body rests on them.

In a variant of this posture, the so called *eight limb salute posture (sāshtānga pranipatāsana)*, the body is brought further down so that it touches the ground at eight – two feet, two palms, two knees, chest, and forehead – points. This is the traditional way an Indian prostrates before the God or elders and hence the name.

7. The Cobra posture (*Bhujangāsana*)

This posture starts with the *stick posture* explained above. Slowly straighten the arms, lift the trunk up and bend it backwards.

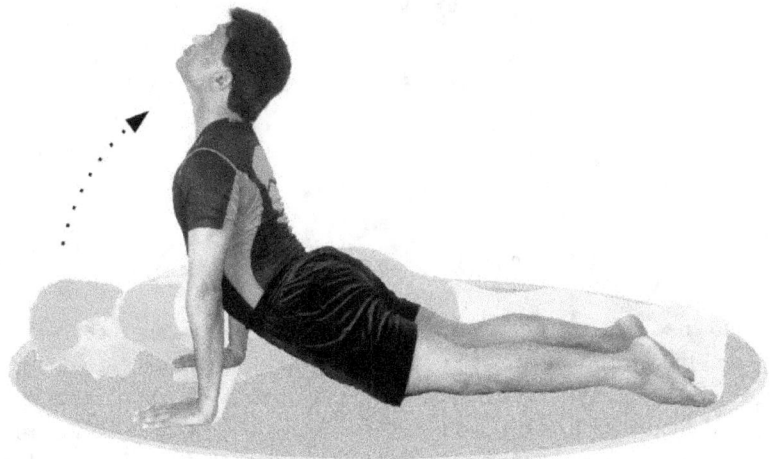

Figure 4.7 Cobra posture (Image courtesy Dr. Omkar)

Stretch the neck backwards and look upwards. Keep the legs stretched. The resulting posture resembles a cobra with its hood open and ready to attack, and hence the name. The final posture is as shown in Figure 4.7.

Benefits: This posture gives good exercise to the spinal cord, shoulders, elbows and the wrist.

8. The Doggy posture (*Adhomukha shvänäsana*)

The starting posture for this is the *cobra posture* that we discussed above. Slowly turn the head downwards and lift the hips upwards. The legs should be stretched straight and the body should form a triangle with the hips at its apex. The down turned face should be facing the feet as shown in Figure 4.8. The posture resembles a dog with its face turned down and hence the name.

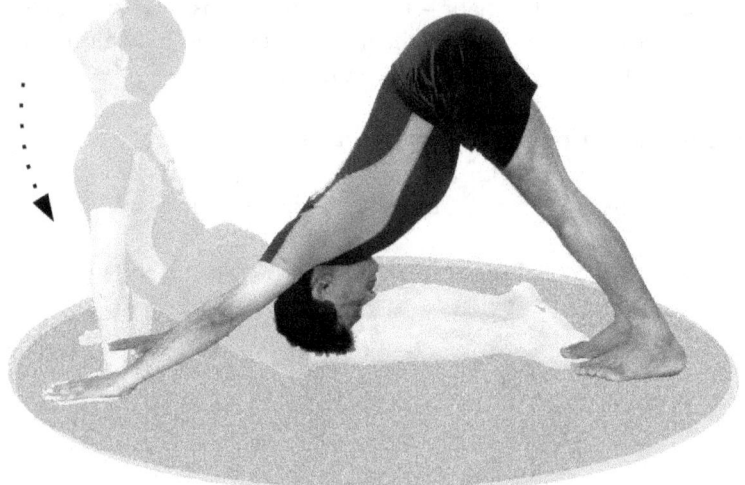

Figure 4.8 Doggy posture (Image courtesy Dr. Omkar)

Benefits: This posture gives a good stretch to the spinal cord. It also strengthens the arms, neck as well as leg muscles.

These 8 simple postures can be performed as they are or can be performed in a cyclical sequence to achieve higher benefit. Let me next give you a stylistic sequencing of these 8 postures – the so called *Sun salutation*.

The Sun salutation (*Suryanamaskära*)

As you probably have noticed, the postures described above seem to transition from one posture to another. This transition is not accidental but intentionally introduced so that these postures can be stitched together to form a nice sequence of postures. This sequence is what is commonly referred to as *Sun salutation*. This sequence combines body postures with controlled breathing (Pränäyäma) as described below.

Sequencing of postures

The sequencing of postures is chosen in such a way that at every stage the muscles are alternatively stretched and de-stretched/compressed. More specifically, the abdominal and the chest muscles are stretched and compressed alternatively. This not only gives good exercise to these muscles and the internal organs, but also aides in controlled breathing.

There are 10 stages in this sequence. The postures are as follows, done back to back in the order listed below.

1. Folded palms posture
2. Backward bend posture
3. Forward bend posture
4. One leg stretch posture
5. Both legs stretch posture
6. Stick posture
7. Cobra posture
8. Doggy posture
9. One leg stretch posture (with alternate leg)
10. Forward bend posture

This sequence can also be viewed as a way of moving the body from a vertical position to a horizontal position (forward) and again back to vertical position (reverse), passing through various intermediate positions. After these 10 postures, the sequence repeats once again with the folded palms posture as shown in Figure 4.9.

Some variants of sun salutations have 12 stages in the sequence as a result of splitting some of the postures into two. But the basic idea is the same.

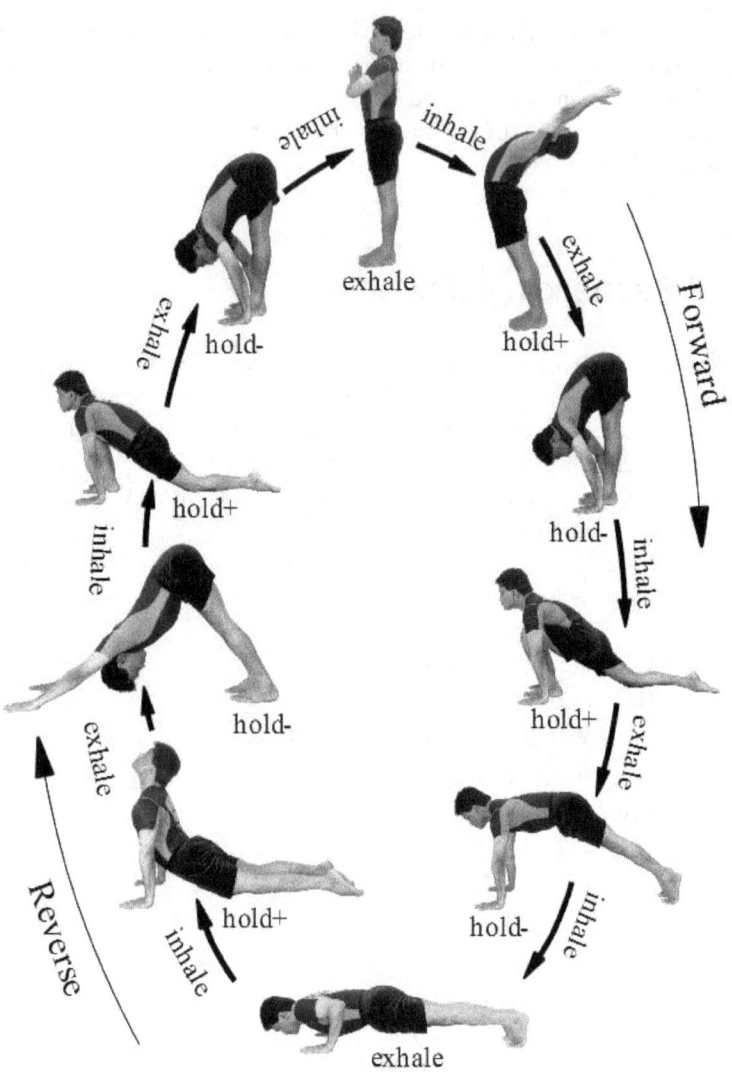

Figure 4.9 Different stages of Sun salutation

Combining the sequence with controlled breathing

Controlled breathing (*Pränäyäma*) is one of the most important aspects of Yoga. I will discuss more on that in Chapter 5. In this section, I will restrict myself to explaining how controlled breathing is combined with various postures of *Sun salutation*.

Our normal breathing has two steps – inhalation and exhalation. Yoga adds two more in between steps that basically involve holding the breath. Accordingly, there are 4 steps in Yogic breathing.

1. Inhale (*Pooraka*) : Take air into the lungs.
2. Hold+ (*Kumbhaka*) : Hold the breath, with lungs filled with air. In Figure 4.9 I have indicted this as **hold+**.
3. Exhale (*Recaka*) : Expel air from the lungs.
4. Hold- (*Shoonyaka*) : Hold the breath, with lungs empty. In Figure 4.9 I have indicted this as **hold-**.

Normally, the duration of hold is much shorter as compared to inhale or exhale.

While combining controlled breathing with the Yoga postures, the general rule of thumb is

*   Inhale if you are reaching a posture by stretching the abdominal and chest muscles.
*   Exhale if you are reaching a posture by compressing the abdominal and chest muscles.
*   Hold+ during a posture if you have reached that posture after inhalation.
*   Hold- during a posture if you have reached that posture after exhalation.

This is clearly shown in Figure 4.9.

Combining faith aspects with *Sun salutation*

Interestingly, *Sun salutation* combines faith aspects (*Īśvara pranidāna* that we discussed in Chapter 2) with the entire sequence. As the name itself indicates, the sequence is about saluting the Sun.

Hindus consider Sun as a visible manifestation of God since Sun is the source of our planet and of all life forms on this planet; it is also the one that nourishes all life forms, and probably one day our planet perishes into the Sun. These three aspects of God namely creation, nourishing and final re-absorption is a criteria common to the definition of God in most religions whether it is Vedic, Biblical or Quranic. Accordingly, Sun is viewed as visible symbol of God.

Normally, Sun *salutations* are performed facing the rising Sun if convenient, or facing east. Facing the rising Sun can have some health benefits as well, due to exposure to mild Sun rays. Alternatively, a devout Christian can probably perform it in front of an image of Jesus Christ, a devout Muslim facing the Kaba, and so on.

As I discussed in Chapter 2, this faith aspect can have its own positive benefits, especially if you are a religiously minded person. Some schools even recommend mentally chanting hymns in praise of Sun.

Some numbers

Normally, multiple cycles of *Sun salutation* are performed at a time. It may take around 15 to 20 seconds to perform one cycle (assuming that you have mastered the postures and the associated breathing regime). That means you can perform 3 to 4 cycles per minute. If you count in terms of the number of controlled breathings you do in each cycle, you will be doing around 6 complete breathings. That means you will be performing around 18 to 24 controlled breathings per minute. This is reasonably a good natural breathing rate.

10 minutes of practice that involves around 30 to 40 *Sun salutation* cycles and 180 to 240 controlled breathings should be good enough. The best practice is to increase the cycle time – that means slow pace of postures and breathing - rather than increasing the cycle count by compressing the cycle time. That way, the mind would become cal-

mer and better effect is attained.

For beginners, it may not be possible to strictly follow the breathing regime indicated in Figure 4.9, especially to remain in hold+ or hold- states. Till one becomes comfortable, it is Ok to take a breath or two before proceeding to the next posture. Also, don't aim for longer practice duration. Pick the pace and duration convenient to you. The postures may look simple, but continuous *Sun salutation* for a prolonged duration can be quite strenuous. So, don't overdo it.

Let me now explain one more posture which is considered to be a whole body exercise as the name itself suggests.

The All limbs posture (*Sarvängäsana*)

Most Yoga teachers laud this posture as the Queen of Yoga postures since it gives exercise to the whole body. This posture is relatively easy but I would advise caution to learn it under the supervision of an experienced teacher, since it involves a slightly unstable inverted posture. Also, since this posture involves inverting the normal upright position of the body, it is said that people with high B.P. and other related problems may experience problems. So seek the advice of your doctor before attempting this posture.

This posture is a multi-stage posture involving 3 distinct intermediate stages before the final one. Different teachers suggest slightly different ways of performing each of these stages. I have shown one such alternative ways. Let me explain these stages one by one.

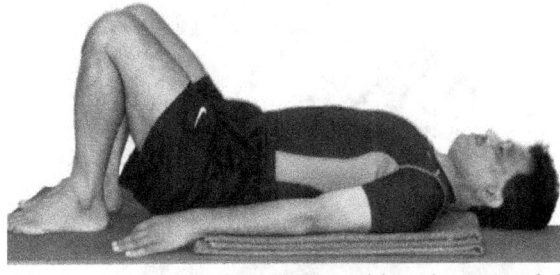

Figure 4.10 All limbs posture - stage 1 (Image courtesy Dr. Omkar)

Stage 1: In this stage, lie down on your back with the head touching the ground, hands stretched on either side of your body, and the legs folded, as shown in Figure 4.10. The folded blanket placed under the back is not essential, but some teachers suggest this to provide some support.

Alternative ways of this stage suggest stretching the legs in line with rest of the body.

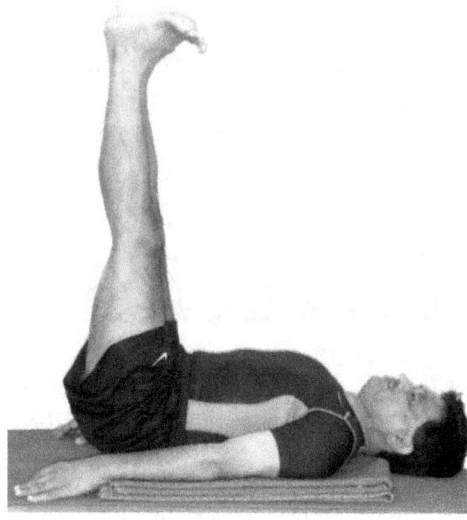

Figure 4.11 All limbs posture - stage 2 (Image courtesy Dr. Omkar)

Stage 2 This is the second stage of the posture. Inhale while you gradually unfold both the legs and stretch them vertically up, so that they are at 90 degrees to the body as shown in Figure 4.11. Keep the hands and the rest of the body as before.

Stage 3
In this third stage of the posture, gradually lift the hips by supporting the back with both the hands as shown in Figure 4.12.

Figure 4.12 All limbs posture - stage 3 (Image courtesy Dr. Omkar)

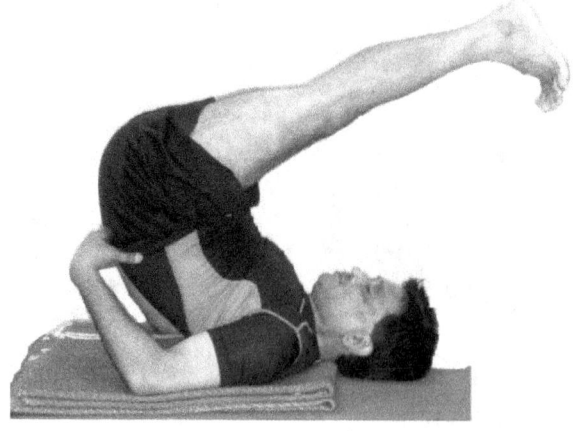

Exhale while doing this. The body weight will be more and more on the shoulders and the arms at this time. Take care not to lose balance and strain your waist or the neck.

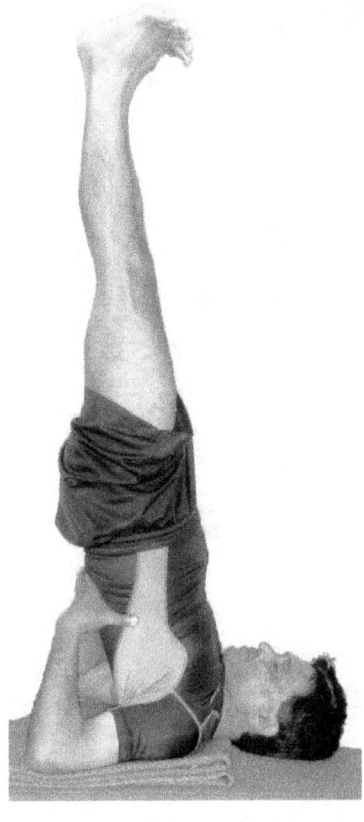

Stage 4

In the next and final stage, while inhaling, raise the back further up with the help of the hands, with the legs stretched straight upwards. In this position, the legs, waist and the back will all be in a straight line perpendicular to the floor. The whole weight of the body will be on the shoulders as well as the upper arms. The chin should be pressing the chest as shown in Figure 4.13.

Figure 4.13 All limbs posture - stage 4
(Image courtesy Dr. Omkar)

You can stay in this final stage as long as you are comfortable – may be a few minutes. During that time breathe normally.

After remaining in the final stage for some time, gradually return back to the stage 1 posture by performing the intermediate postures in the reverse order as shown in Figure 4.14. This figure shows both the forward as well as the reverse stages along with associated breathing regime.

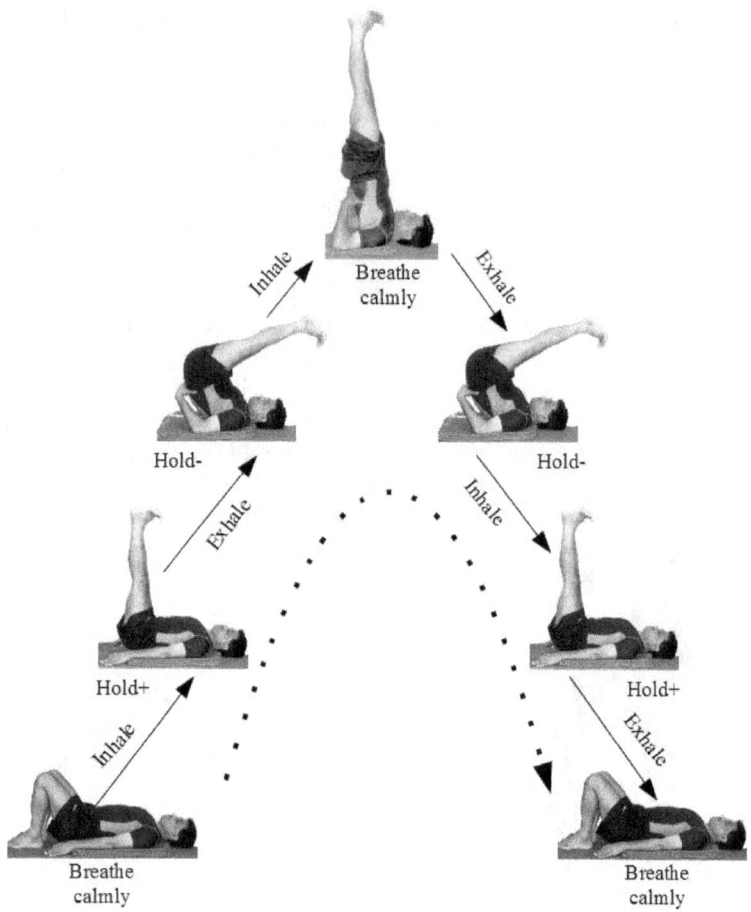

Figure 4.14 All limbs posture – complete sequence

Benefits: Whole lots of benefits are attributed to this *all limbs posture* apart from giving exercise to entire body. Some of the claimed benefits include

- This posture gives good exercise to the spine, neck, and shoulder blades.
- The thyroid glands get good stimulation.
- This helps in minimizing headaches and migraines.
- This posture is supposed to reduce loss of hair and premature graying of hair.

- This may help in eye, nose and throat ailments.

- This is beneficial for people suffering from indigestion, constipation.

- Due to this inverted posture, the valves of the blood vessels receive a negative blood pressure clearing any blockage or mal-function.

- Beneficial in the case of many problems relating to the reproductory systems.

In the foregoing chapters we saw how we can free ourselves from mental stress as well as how we can keep our body healthy. A healthy body with a stress free mind is definitely what one can ask for. But to enjoy life, we need to use them gainfully. After all, these are just pre-requisites for success in life.

All of us would like to accomplish lot of things in life. For doing that, we need to apply our mind to whatever we want to achieve in our life. Most of the time we fail to do that due to lack of focus. Needless to say that a focused mind free of stress and residing in a healthy body, can achieve miracles.

In the next chapter I am going to discuss this important aspect and how Yoga can help us in cultivating a focused mind.

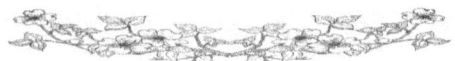

5 A focused mind can achieve miracles

In the previous chapters, we discussed how one can develop a sound mind as well as a sound body by following the processes enlisted in Yoga. Good physical as well as mental health is essential for peaceful living. But is that all? Many people with sound body and mind fail to perform well in life. Most of the time the primary cause is poor focus, whether it is the clarity on what one wants to achieve or most importantly due to poor concentration on whatever one does.

Many students experience lot of difficulty in their studies even though they sincerely try to study. I have seen students who spend hours reading their books but very little is absorbed and remembered. The prominent cause for this is what is generally termed as mind wandering. Our mind generally tends to wander away from the task on hand. So the necessary attention required to perform a task is not paid adequately. Needless to say that this can have adverse consequences on the quality of the task performed.

This applies not only to students but also to any person. A person, no matter what profession he follows, performs poorly if he does not pay necessary attention to whatever he is doing, in spite of the fact that he is physically and mentally sound. In other words, poor concentration can result in inefficient deployment of physical and mental resources and ultimately in mediocre performance. Conversely, any task performed by paying full attention can excel in all respects.

It is possible to train the mind for better focus

Barring some pathological conditions, it is possible for a normal person to sharpen his ability to focus on the task of interest. Yoga has techniques to do this. These techniques may not increase our mental resources but will definitely result in their better utilization.

The cause of poor concentration

As I said above, the primary cause is the mind wandering. Our mind continuously generates thoughts that may or may not be related to the tasks that we perform at any time. These thoughts contend for brain resources, effectively diverting the resources needed for the task on hand. Obviously this ends up in poor performance.

In Part I of this series, I have explained how the attention system, mainly rooted in the thalamus, effectively coordinates the sharing of information between various neural network assemblies spread across the brain. Thoughts too utilize this system. Too many task unrelated thoughts result in overload on this attention system due to rapid switching of attention.

In the best case, this rapid switching may delay useful task related processes since they are kept waiting. In the worst case, these useful processes may gradually die down since the neural networks supporting those processes do not get the necessary activity boosting that is usually provided by the attention system. In Part I we have seen how this can happen. In both cases, the performance of the task of interest suffers.

How do we improve focus or concentration?

The attention system in our brain, like any other brain functional unit, is made up of neural networks. So it should be possible to train these neural networks in such a way that they are biased more towards the thoughts related to the task of interest rather than to the thoughts that are not related. When this happens, the task related thoughts get an upper hand, and can utilize the brain resources more effectively. At the same time, the task unrelated thoughts gradually die down due to lack of attention. We don't fully understand how training of the attention system works, but definitely there are Yoga as well as other techniques that help us in achieving that. In this chapter, I will discuss some of them.

Some simple techniques to improve concentration

In this section, I will discuss some simple techniques that can potentially improve our concentration. These techniques picked from Yoga as well as other related disciplines, need minimal resources, and may internally work in a similar manner. What is all the more interesting is that some of these techniques can potentially take us towards the ultimate goals of Yoga as we discuss in Chapter 6. Let me start with a simple Yoga technique.

Controlled breathing (*Pränäyäma*)

We have already talked about controlled breathing in the context of *Sun salutation* that we discussed in Chapter 4. Patanjali calls it *Pränäyäma*. This breathing essentially has four components – inhalation, holding the breath (with lungs full), exhalation, and holding the breath (with empty lungs). Patanjali talks about variations in these breathing steps in terms of duration of each step.

For our purpose, we can decide on the duration of each of these steps based on our comfort and gradually try to increase this duration. All that one needs to do is to consciously breathe in at a convenient pace, hold the breath for a convenient duration, breath out at a convenient pace and finally hold the breath for a convenient duration. Though not essential, you can use your fingers to open and close the nose and guide the inhalation and exhalation.

Repeat this cycle of breathing consciously for some time. Gradually increase the duration of each step, and the total number of controlled breathing cycles, once you are comfortable with this practice. This is the simplest form of controlled breathing.

This controlled breathing can be clubbed with different stages of a specific Yoga posture or sequence of postures. We have already seen how this is done in Chapter 4. More importantly, it can be practiced as a standalone technique for the sole purpose of improving the concentration.

If done in the latter fashion, it is advisable for the person to sit in a comfortable posture in a calm place and do the practice for certain duration. The suitable posture can be any of the postures discussed in Chapter 6. However, doing it for a prolonged duration, say several tens of minutes at a time, may have its adverse effects that I will talk about later in this section.

Why does it work?

We don't as of now know how exactly this breathing exercise improves concentration. The fact is that it does. The reason could be as follows. Breathing is one of our essential bodily activities needed for survival. Though breathing is a semiautonomous activity, we can willingly stop it or play with it, at least for some time. But stopping it is life threatening and hence the body has automatic mechanisms to divert the attention to whatever that caused the stoppage of this essential activity. Hold your breath for some time and try to simultaneously think of anything that interests you the most – may be about your lover! You can't do it. Your attention will be all concentrated on the suffocation caused by holding of breath.

Probably, this is what happens when you do controlled breathing. The restriction put on the natural flow of breath automatically forces the attention system to ignore any other activity that may try to draw its attention. Repeated practice of this controlled breathing probably trains the attention system to pay attention to one and only one high priority activity rather than get diverted to several contending ones.

Alternate schools of Yoga have various mysterious explanations about why controlled breathing works and how it can have miraculous effects on the practitioner. Accordingly, they have rigid rules on the specific nostril through which the air has to be drawn in and expelled out, several ways of doing it, and so on. Each of these ways is supposed to have some special effect on the practitioner and his *subtle body*. However, neither Patanjali, nor his commentator Vyāsa talk anything about them. In this book, I will restrict myself to breathing techniques, whose working can be explained in a logical way.

Let me next discuss another breathing related technique taken from the Buddhist school.

Mindful breathing (*Änäpäna sati*)

Sati is a class of Buddhist techniques useful in focusing the mind. The *Pali* (an ancient language) word *sati* is often translated as mindfulness or doing something with full concentration. These techniques are explained in *Satipatthana Sutta* of *Suttapitaka*, which in turn is a part of *Tipitaka* - the earliest (~300 B.C.) recordings of Buddha's teachings. I have discussed more on *Tipitaka* in Part II of this series.

Änäpäna sati is considered to be one of the most important *sati* techniques. The word *Änäpäna* means inhalation and exhalation. So it is a technique involving breathing in and out. The way it is done is slightly different from the Yogic one. Here, there is no conscious control of the breath, but merely monitoring the natural breathing process in a dispassionate way.

Just observe how the air moves in, how it fills the lungs, how it gets expelled out, how the lungs get emptied, and how there is a pause before the cycle repeats. Focus your attention fully on this natural process of breathing and nothing else.

Buddhist schools claim that just this technique can take one to the highest levels of Buddhist meditation. In fact, it is claimed that

Buddha attained his final enlightenment just by practicing this technique.

Though the techniques of *Pränäyäma* and *Änäpäna* sati differ in the details, they seem to internally work the same way.

Let me next explain one more focusing technique taken from alternate schools of Yoga.

Candle gazing (*Trätaka*)

This is yet another practice meant to improve concentration. This is not part of Patanjali Yoga. However, some variants of Yoga talk about this practice. For example, the *Hatayoga Pradeepika* talks briefly about it.

The technique is quite simple. Just sit in a comfortable posture in front of a lighted candle as shown in Figure 5.1. The place where you do this practice should be free from strong gusts of wind that can make the candle flame unsteady. The candle flame should be at the same level as your eyes, as shown in the figure. The distance between your eyes and the candle flame can be chosen in such a way that it does not put unnecessary strain on your eyes.

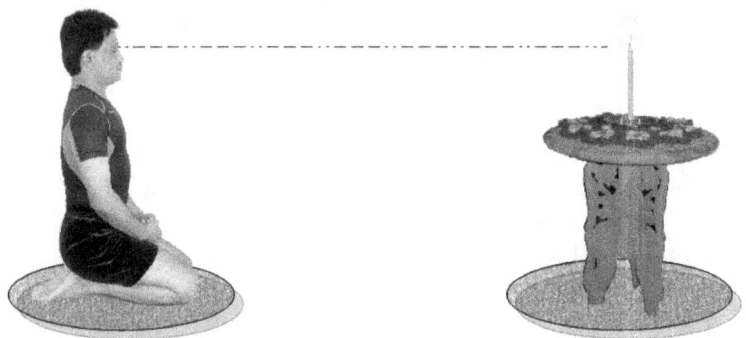

Figure 5.1 Trätaka or candle gazing to improve concentration

Keep staring at the flame without blinking your eyelids as long as you can comfortably do it. When your eyes are tired, close them for a while and give them some rest. Repeat the process again. Do this for say, some 10 minutes. While staring at the flame, try to remain calm and relaxed. Also, as far as possible try to focus your attention on the flame, its shape, color, and so on.

Some modern schools provide an electronic version, with a small LED lit behind a plastic enclosure and its light emanating from a pin hole in the enclosure. This may be more convenient to use since there is no hassle of the flame swaying due to wind. But using a candle flame may be more effective. Again, prolonged practice of just this technique alone, can take one to higher levels of Yoga practice.

It is said that this practice can strengthen eye muscles and probably help in overcoming eye problems. However, use caution not to over exert your eyes.

Let me next talk about another interesting technique, namely mantra chanting, that has been in use for thousands of years for focusing the mind.

Mantra chanting

Whether it is controlled breathing, mindful breathing or candle gazing, the end result is a sharply focused mind: the mind focused on one and only one task at a given time. Such sharpness in focus can be good if one wants to continue with Yoga and get on to the stages of meditation and so on. It may also be good for people whose profession needs keen focus, like scientists and the like.

But most of the jobs performed by 'normal' people involves multi-tasking. That is, a person is expected to do more than one task at a given time. The person keeps switching between a limited set of tasks that are of interest and would like to attain perfection, or at least near perfection, in each of the tasks. A highly focused mind tends to get stuck in one task, however perfectly it executes it.

So, what is normally required is a good balance between focus and the ability to willingly switch between multiple tasks. This is the normal requirement for most people dealing with the world around. How does one train the attention system to sharpen its ability to focus, and at the same time retain its ability to switch between a small set of tasks that are of interest.

Chanting some specially designed Mantras is believed to achieve this. In general, a mantra is just a sound or a sequence of sounds with or without meaning. Different mantras are supposed to have different effects on our mind. I have discussed about one mantra in my book **"A Mantra to enhance your Mental Capabilities"** that is specially meant for improving the concentration as well as in enabling one to do multi-tasking in a controlled fashion.

This mantra with thousands of years of history has been in use even today in India. It is basically administered to students at the time of their joining formal schools. The purpose of administering this mantra is clearly stated in ancient scriptures - for sharpening the concentration as well as the mental capability of the student. The student is expected to chant this mantra in a pre-specified manner every day without fail.

I will not go into the details of that mantra here (you may refer to the above mentioned book), but merely try to explain how the mantra probably achieves these claimed benefits.

How does the mantra work?

What is done in mantra chanting is that the mantra is repeated either audibly or mentally. During the chanting, the mind is focused on the sound variations that occur while the mantra is being chanted. The mantra I discussed in the above mentioned book has the sound pattern shown in Figure 5.2.

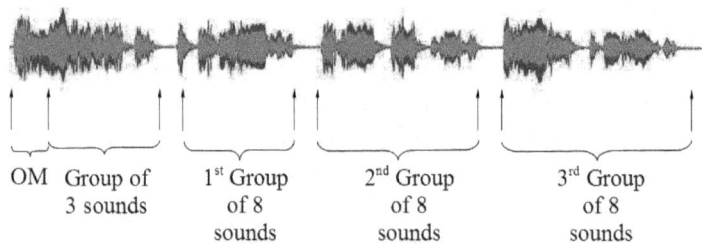

| OM | Group of 3 sounds | 1st Group of 8 sounds | 2nd Group of 8 sounds | 3rd Group of 8 sounds |

Figure 5.2 Variation in sound in the mantra

The part indicated as 'OM' itself is considered to be a mantra when chanted on its own. It has its own effects on the mind, which I am going to discuss more in Chapter 6. Basically, it is supposed to calm the mind. So, traditionally, it is a practice to prefix OM before any mantra so that the mantra that follows is chanted with a calm mind and the mind is more receptive to its effects.

The prominent component of this mantra is a set of 3 groups of 8 sounds each, as shown in Figure 5.2. If you notice carefully, in each of these 3 groups, there is some regularity of sounds, while there is also some gradual variation. This variation is not monotonic. The sound intensity increases and decreases rather abruptly. Probably it is this regularity combined with variations is what gives this mantra the capability to achieve the required effect.

When attention is focused on this sound sequence, the mind not only gets well focused but also not oblivious to changes that are part of the sound sequence. So there is an attempt to balance between absolute concentration, and the capability to take note of changes and adapt to it.

However, it should be noted that prolonged chanting of this mantra, say for hours at a time, would make the mind more engrossed and focused. So, it is normally advised not to chant the mantra more than 100 times at a time. It takes roughly 20 minutes to chant the mantra 100 times and that is also the duration needed for the attention system to get trained, as observed in some scientific experiments.

There are some questions to which probably we don't have precise answers. Why 3 groups of exactly 8 sounds? Why the choice of a specific set of sounds? And so on. It should be remembered that this mantra is not just a set of sounds. It has lot of religious connotation and meaning associated with each group of sounds. You can refer to **"A Mantra to enhance your Mental Capabilities"** for these details and instructions on how to chant this mantra.

Briefly, the meaning associated with this mantra is a prayer to a very broad definition of God to stimulate intellect. Whether this meaning and the associated religious connotation, are meant to induce a conducive mental makeup, we do not know.

Dual role of these techniques

The techniques discussed so far have dual role. Their primary role is to train the attention system so that it is either completely focused, or focused but still capable of multi-tasking. At the same time, these techniques calm the mind due to minimization of unnecessary thoughts and switching of attention. So they work as powerful stress minimizers.

One can practice these techniques either for improving the focus or for the sole purpose of stress minimization. The latter is the effect that is mainly achieved when controlled breathing is clubbed with Yoga postures.

However, if practiced for a prolonged duration they work more as meditation which I am going to discuss in the next chapter. Unless that is what is intended, it is advisable not to practice these techniques for more than few tens of minutes at a time.

Improving physical health, minimizing stress, and developing a focused mind are definitely the things everyone would like to achieve. Yoga helps in realizing each of these. But the real aim of Yoga is to completely quieten the mind so that we can 'realize' our true identity that is often masked when the mind is engrossed in worldly activities. That is what can potentially give us lasting peace. How we go about doing that, is what I am going to discuss next.

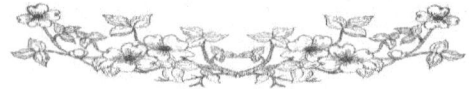

6 Shutting off the unruly ghost

In the last few chapters we saw how some of the processes of Yoga are performed, and how they help us in enjoying a healthy and stress free life. We also discussed how we can improve our focus so that we can realize our full mental potential. Let me briefly summarize what we have seen so far, and put that in the proper perspective in the broader context of Yoga.

In Chapter 2, we discussed how we can block the causes of stress by following a specific life style. This is the first step of the eight-step Yoga. Yoga calls this step as *Yama*. Minimization of the causes of stress results in minimizing the negative thoughts – the major contributors to stress.

Simultaneously, we can fortify positive thoughts by developing a positive frame of mind. This is the second step and is called *Niyama*. We discussed this step, also in Chapter 2. Together, these two steps relieve us from stress to a large extent. As we saw in Chapter 1, minimization of stress can in all probability reduce the chances of our falling ill.

We also saw a completely alternate way of overcoming stress through devotional singing in Chapter 3. This practice has some overlap with the *Īswara Pranidāna* suggested by Yoga. This approach is very natural and easy to follow, for most of us.

In Chapter 4, we saw how by practicing certain body postures we can strengthen our body and remain healthy. This is the 3rd step of Yoga. Yoga calls it *asana*, though the body postures we discussed go beyond the basic definition of *asana* and have their roots in later variants of Yoga.

A healthy body and mind is not good enough unless we are also able to focus on our chosen professions and achieve success in our lives. In Chapter 5, I suggested some Yoga as well as non Yoga techniques using which we can sharpen our focusing skills. The Yogic technique called *Pränäyäma* is one of these techniques, and it forms the 4th step of Yoga.

In essence, in these chapters we covered the first four of the eight steps of Yoga, namely *Yama*, *Niyama*, *Asana* and *Pränäyäma* as shown in Figure 6.1. That means, we are only half way through.

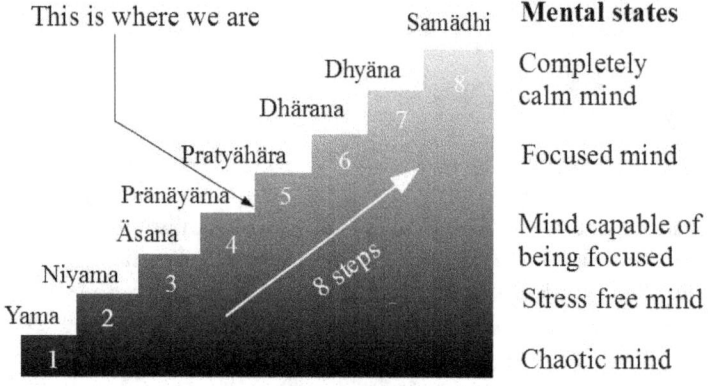

Figure 6.1 Eight steps of Yoga

If you are a person content with living a 'normal' worldly life, with a sound mind and a body, almost free from stress, doing your job to the best of your capabilities, you can stop at this stage. It is like the way one progresses during his student life.

When you are pursuing your studies, you have a choice to drop out at high school level, take-up some job and somehow manage to live; or you can continue your studies, complete graduation, take up a good job and make a good comfortable living. You can choose to go further, spend several years of dedicated toiling, get a Ph.D. and not only have the satisfaction of having achieved something, but also live comfortably, earning lot of respect in the society. Choice is yours.

Probably, most would continue till graduation and very few dedicated ones proceed further and complete their Ph.D. The reward they get cannot be measured in terms of worldly benefits. It is something higher than that.

So also, higher levels of Yoga practice that I am going to discuss in this chapter demand greater dedication and effort, may rob you off some of your worldly comforts, may not mean much in mundane terms, but all the same, worth trying.

The steps you have seen in the previous chapters are like completing the graduation and earning the eligibility to take up Ph.D. If you choose to continue with the processes that I discuss in the following sections, you will be rewarded with higher levels of mental calmness and also a glimpse of the things that are beyond the realms of mind. Let us move on.

The real goal of Yoga is to completely calm the mind

Whatever goals we discussed in previous chapters are not the 'real' goals of Yoga but only byproducts. Unfortunately, many schools tend to overemphasize and project them as the real goals of Yoga. As Patanjali (Yoga Sutra 1.2) says

Yoga is about restraining the activities of the mind.

By restraining he means completely calming down the mind. Patanjali also lists (Yoga Sutra 2.2) attaining *samädhi* and minimizing the effects of *Kleshas* as the purpose of Yoga.

(This Yoga) is meant for attainment of samädhi and minimization of the effects of Kleshas.

I will discuss about *samädhi* later in this chapter and about *Kleshas* in the next chapter. Basically, *samädhi* is a completely calm state of the mind and *Kleshas* are the preset imprints on the mind that put us into an endless cycle of miseries.

You probably think that the Yoga processes that we discussed in the previous chapters have already enabled us in achieving a calm mind. Not really so. What we have really achieved so far is to bring the mind from a near chaotic condition to a state that is capable of being focused (refer to Figure 6.1). Making it completely calm is a long call and that is the topic of this chapter.

Why is it difficult to calm the mind completely?

Just imagine sitting for a moment without any thoughts in your mind. It is almost impossible. More you try, more thoughts get generated and you need to put more effort. Our mind is like the mythical ghost that keeps doing something all the time and it is beyond our control. That is why I call it 'unruly ghost'. How do we quieten this unruly ghost namely the mind? It can't be done by force. Yoga has a better way. Obviously, that way is through meditation.

Meditation is the Yoga way to calm the mind

In Chapter 5, we saw how we can train our attention system to focus on any given object. Having sharpened our focusing skills, we need to focus the mind on some object, which I am going to discuss soon. Yoga calls this process as *Dhārana*. This is the 6th step of Yoga as shown in Figure 6.1. Continuously keeping the mind focused on the chosen object is meditation or *Dhyāna* as Yoga calls it. Meditation is the penultimate step of Yoga.

Meditation can be a long process that may need one to remain in a given posture for prolonged duration of time – from tens of minutes to even hours. There are some postures that are ideally suited for such long duration of practice. Let me now explain some of the postures that may be useful for the purpose of meditation.

Some useful body postures for meditation

Probably, the easiest posture for most of us is to just lie down. Surprisingly, even this seemingly trivial posture is a Yoga posture called the 'corpse posture' (*Shavāsana*), useful for complete relaxation after rigorous workout. But the problem with this posture is that we tend to fall asleep when we put ourselves in that posture since our body is conditioned that way. So, we need a posture that does not make us fall asleep. There are also other requirements for a good meditative posture as we will see further on. One of the most recommended meditative postures is what is called the *lotus posture* or the *Padmäsana*.

The Lotus posture (*Padmäsana*)

This is the best posture suitable for prolonged duration of meditation. Figure 6.2 shows how one can sit in this posture. To sit in this posture

1. Sit on the floor with both legs stretched out.

2. Now hold the left foot with one hand and gradually move it up in such a way that it is finally placed on the right thigh with the heel touching the lower abdomen.

3. Similarly, place the right foot on the left thigh with the heel touching the lower abdomen. In this position the lower legs would be crossing each other as shown in Figure 6.2 . The feet would be opening up like a blooming lotus. Hence this asana is called the *lotus posture*.

4. Keep the back and neck straight.

5. Keep the palms locked and placed at the junction of the crossed legs as shown in Figure 6.2.

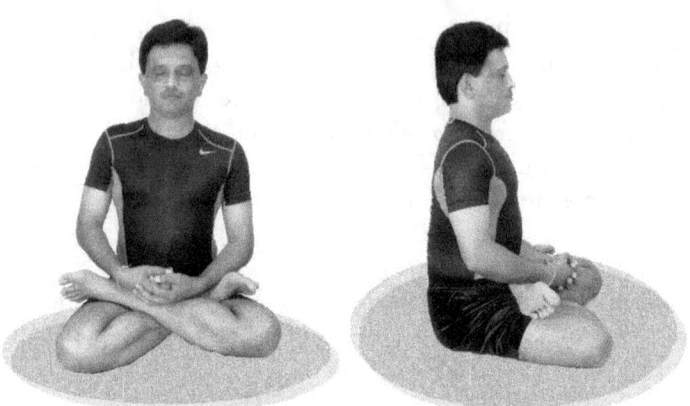

Figure 6.2 The Lotus posture (Image courtesy Dr. Omkar)

This asana gives stability to the body during prolonged meditation. Without this stability

- The body may tremble when the mind is focused on the chosen object, since the required attention is not paid to the body. This trembling may distract the mind from focus and hinder meditation.

- At advanced stages of meditation, when one enters the state of *samādhi*, the body may collapse due to lack of control. The way the legs and the hands are locked in this posture provides the necessary mechanical stability to the body, preventing it from collapse.

- The body may tend to fall asleep during meditation. But we need to be alert all through. The locked legs help us in keeping the back and neck straight. Also, the locked legs prevent leaning forward, the tendency that normally occurs while falling asleep.

Adept Yoga practitioners say that once you master this posture, it is not only stable but comfortable as well, meeting both the requirements of asana as specified by Patanjali. Just to recall, the very definition of asana given by Patanjali (Yoga Sutra, 2.46) is

Asana is that which is stable and comfortable

However, not all may be able to sit in this posture. Especially, if your knee joints are not flexible enough, it can be quite painful. Even when you are able to lift the legs and cross them as shown, you may need to practice it for several days before you can sit exactly as shown.

In any case, don't force yourselves. Otherwise there is a chance that you may injure your knees. For those of you who find the *lotus posture* difficult, the next best alternative is the so called *comfortable posture*.

The comfortable posture (*Sukhāsana* or *Svastikāsana*)

As the name indicates, this one is relatively a comfortable posture. This posture is almost similar to the *lotus posture*. But you don't need to lift the heels and place them on the thighs as in *lotus posture*. But the back and neck have to be straight as before. Also, the palms should be locked and placed at the junction of the crossed legs.

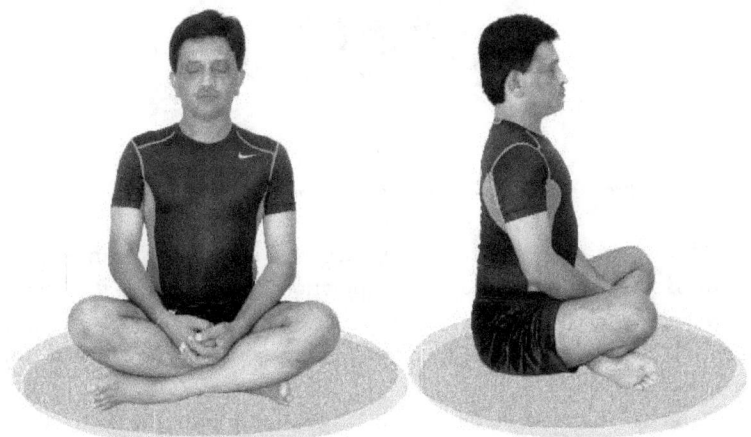

Figure 6.3 The comfortable posture (Image courtesy Dr. Omkar)

This posture is the most natural posture for most eastern cultures since this is the posture in which they sit while praying, discussing or even while dining. This has the advantage of comfort, while the stability aspect is slightly compromised.

Some westerners may find even crossing the legs difficult. For them the next best is what we have already seen in Figure 5.1, namely the *Diamond posture*.

The Diamond posture (*Vajräsana*)

This posture is as shown in Figure 6.4. Except for the legs, rest of the limbs are as in *lotus posture* or the *comfortable posture* – the back and neck straight, the palms locked and kept on the leg junction.

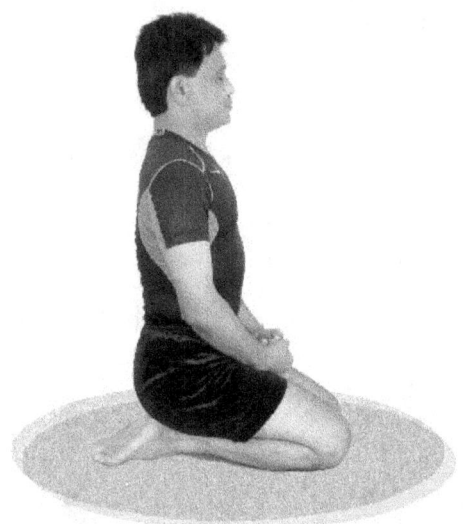

Figure 6.4 The Diamond posture (Image courtesy Dr. Omkar)

All these postures have varying degrees of difficulty in mastering them. Before you start the regular practice of meditation, it is better to master one of these postures depending on your comfort. This may take concerted attempts spanning several days. Be cautious and progress carefully.

After mastering a suitable meditative posture, the next step is to choose an object to focus on. The choice of this object depends on the mental makeup of the person and convenience. Some of these are considered to be the best, and others are next best choices as I explain below.

Objects to focus on

The objects for focus can be either gross or subtle. By gross object I mean the objects that can be either seen with the eyes or heard with the ears and so on, i.e. some external object that can be perceived through our senses.

It could be the image of your favorite deity, or some religious symbol, or a lit candle as in candle gazing that we discussed in Chapter 5, the sound produced by chanting of some mantra, sound of a bell or some such device, and so on.

Some people may be puzzled when I suggest some visible object as an object of focus for meditation, since many think that meditation is always with eyes closed. That is not so. Many Buddhist schools recommend meditation with eyes partially open. Open so that one does not fall asleep; partially open so that one does not get distracted by things that are going on around. Even the *Bhagavad Geetha* recommends staring at the tip of one's nose while meditating!

There is one object – audible- that is considered to be the best meditative focus. That is the so called 'Pranava Mantra' or the *OM* sound as it is usually referred to. Even Patanjali recommends this as the best object for meditation. *Upanishads* and most ancient Indian texts suggest this as the best target for meditation. Even the Buddhists and other supposed adversaries of Vedic school also use this sound for meditation. So let me talk a bit more in detail about this most favored object of focus during meditation.

The OM sound as the focus of meditation

The *OM* sound is just the sound produced when you utter the two letters 'O' and "M" together in a particular way. In Sanskrit, when these two letters are uttered together, they are considered to be a single letter namely *OM*. Lot has been talked about this letter in many ancient scriptures. This letter is supposed to be the eternal letter that is supposed to have existed from time immemorial.

The Upanishads identify three sounds merged into one, when one utters *OM*. These sounds are 'A', 'U', and "M" - the sound 'A' as the letter 'u' in the word 'up', the sound 'U' as the letter 'u' in the word 'put', and the sound 'M' as the letter 'm' in the word 'dim'. Various interpretations are given as to what each of these sounds represent and what the combined sound represents. Some of these interpretations may help in providing the necessary mental setting while meditating on this sound.

The sound 'A' is considered to be corresponding to creation, the sound 'U' corresponding to sustenance, and the sound 'M' corresponding to the final re-absorption. In most religions, these three are considered to be the three prominent aspects of God. So *Upanishads* declare *OM* – the sound combining these three sounds – as the definition of God itself. Even Patanjali says (Yoga Sutra 1.27)

> *OM symbolizes him (i.e. God)*

Patanjali further says (Yoga Sutra 1.28)

> *One should meditate on this (i.e. OM) by mentally*
> *visualizing the meaning of this.*

The way this sound *OM* is made is different when it is prefixed to some general mantra, as compared to when it is chanted in a standalone manner as a *Pranava mantra*. The sound pattern of the latter is something like what is shown in Figure 6.5

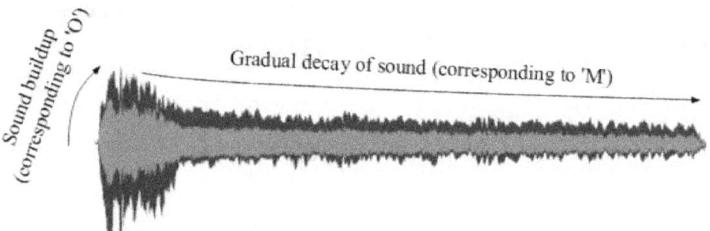

Figure 6.5 Sound variations in Pranava mantra

If you observe your breath while making this sound you can notice that you will be inhaling during the sound buildup time and slowly exhaling during the gradual sound decay time. The length of the gradual decay determines when this sound is made as standalone *Pranava mantra* and when it is made as a prefix to some other mantra.

For example, in Figure 5.2 (where *OM* is used as a prefix), the *OM* abruptly ends – short decay time - since it is immediately succeeded by the three other sounds. This difference in usage has important consequences that I will come to in the next section.

The best practice is to make this *Pranava* sound by chanting it.

Special metal gongs or bells are also available that can produce *Pranava* like sound when struck. These devices are sometimes used for meditative purposes. In Figure 6.6, I have shown a bronze bell specially crafted to emanate *Pranava* like sound. This bell was bought from some Tibetan refugee settlement in India.

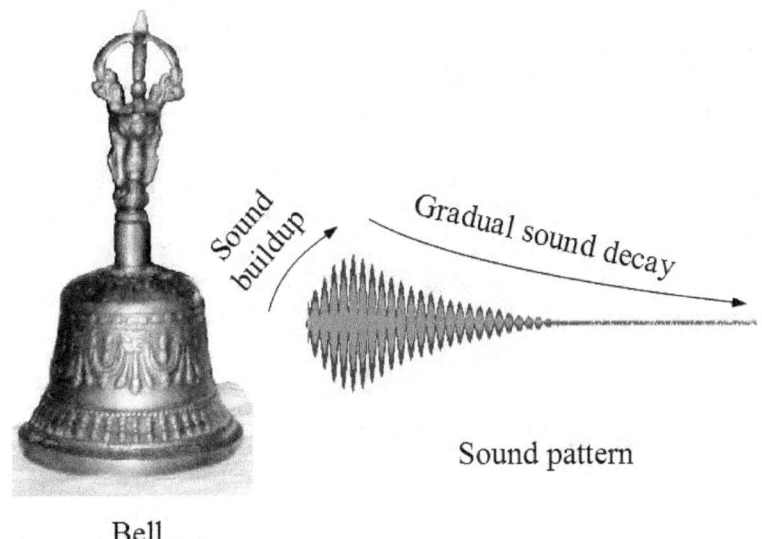

Bell

Sound pattern

Figure 6.6 A bronze bell used to produce Pranava like sound

Compare the shape of the sound wave shown in Figure 6.6 with that shown in Figure 6.5. The one produced by the bell is more clean and perfect in shape. But the vocally produced sound has the advantage of synchronizing the breathing with the sound production.

In modern electronic era, even recorded *Pranava* chanting is used as meditative aide.

External objects as targets of meditation are OK for the beginners. But as one progresses in meditation practice, it is better to focus on mental analogues of these external objects. For example, one can mentally visualize the image of his favorite deity, or visualize a steady candle flame or even mentally chant a mantra and focus the mind on its sound variation and associated breathing rhythm. That would not only avoid distractions from the external world, but also eliminate the inevitable mental activity needed to perceive the external target.

One can start with a gross object, and gradually migrate to subtle objects as one makes progress.

What happens during meditation?

The things that disturb the focus are the external sense inputs or internally generated thoughts. By choosing a quiet secluded environment, external disturbances can be minimized. Interestingly, after some practice, the external disturbances fail to attract attention and go without being noticed even if the eyes, ears, and so on are open. The external sense organs convey the information to the mind, but they fail to get registered and processed. This is what Patanjali calls as *Pratyāhāra*. Though listed as the 5th step of Yoga, it is actually a state that one reaches after some initial meditation practice.

What is *Pratyāhāra*?

As some people wrongly interpret, *Pratyāhāra* is not some special dietary constraint put on the Yoga practitioner. Nor it is about willfully controlling the senses. It is just a state that is reached when someone acquires a focused mind. Patanjali is very clear on this. To quote from Yoga Sutra 2.54,

> *The state when the sense organs don't get involved*
> *in their respective sense inputs is called Pratyāhāra.*

One should remember that Yoga considers sense organs as a combination of external (gross) and internal (subtle) organs. Probably we can interpret *pratyāhāra* as the state when external sense organs continue to process inputs but the parts of the brain that are involved in processing them stop processing. Why they stop processing, we will see next.

Why does the sense perception stop?

It is commonly noticed that when you are seriously engrossed in some thought, you fail to perceive anything that is happening around you, even when your eyes are wide open! Exactly same thing happens when one is focused on some meditative object. The mind refuses to pay attention to the incoming inputs from the sense organs and these inputs gradually die down for lack of attention. This attention is needed for further processing of these sense inputs. The *Yoga Sutra* commentator gives a nice simile to illustrate this *pratyāhāra* state. He says

Like the bees that follow the Queen Bee, so also the senses stop functioning once the mind has stopped functioning (i.e. they just follow the mind)

The commentator further clarifies that this stoppage of sense perception does not need any additional effort. It just happens automatically.

Beyond *Pratyāhāra*

As the meditation continues, we are left with only thoughts that are active in our mind. As I said earlier, thoughts are sporadically produced neural activities that may or may not be related to the task on hand. Our task on hand is the act of continuing focus – meditation - on the chosen object.

But it is possible that initially whole lot of other thoughts totally unrelated to this task can get generated and each of them may not only try to draw the attention, but also try to inhibit the task related thoughts. This results in subtle stress.

As you know, any neural activity can be sustained only if one or more of the following happens

- Stimulation from inputs from the external sense organs
- Support from other related neural activities.
- Boost provided by the attention system.

If none of these happen, then the activity gradually dies down. This dying down not only eliminates the thought but also prevents formation of other cascading thoughts that might spurt from this one. As we saw in the previous section, because of the *Pratyāhāra* state we have reached, external inputs cannot support these thoughts. Since we have trained our attention system to pay attention to only the task on hand – meditation, these task-unrelated thoughts don't get the required attention. So, over a period of time, these task-unrelated thoughts gradually die down.

What happens when all task unrelated thoughts are eliminated?

Reduction of task-unrelated thoughts not only reduces the load on the attention system but also minimizes the conflicts between the two kinds of thoughts – task related and task unrelated. This results in further reduction in stress. The person who meditates experiences bliss when this happens,. This bliss is not because of any sense pleasure, but merely because of lack of anything that prevents bliss.

Bliss without any object that induces the bliss may look surprising. Ask a chronic Asthma patient how he feels when he takes a puff from his inhaler. He feels enjoyment even in the mundane act of breathing. This enjoyment comes from the lack of deterrent to enjoyment!

This is the first stage of *samādhi* where there are task related thoughts and the person experiences bliss due to lack of task unrelated thoughts. Patanjali calls it *Vitarkānugata samādhi*. In this state the mind remains calm, but not completely devoid of any activity, since the task related thoughts are still present.

Before I proceed further, let me touch upon another issue that I postponed while discussing about a specific mantra in Chapter 5. I was talking about why the sound *OM* is prefixed to the mantra that is useful for attaining a focused mind that is still capable of doing multi-tasking.

The reason seems to be that *OM* has the potential to calm the mind for the reasons cited above. A calm mind may make the attention system more receptive to training. However, complete *OM* as recited in the case of the *Pranava mantra* may make the mind so calm that the person may get engrossed in a single task, without being able to do multi-tasking. So to balance out the conflicting requirements of calmness and ability to switch attention across multiple tasks of interest, *OM* is recited partially as a prefix to the mantra. The immediately succeeding 3 sounds abruptly terminate the decaying part (refer to Figure 5.2 and Figure 6.5) of *OM*.

Why are various stages of *samādhi* attained?

Samādhi is a series of final stages of meditation. I have explained in greater detail about various stages of *samādhi* in my book **Psychology behind Yoga**. In that book I have given a conceptual description of how these stages are attained. In this book however, I will try to give a neurologically based explanation about how these stages are attained.

Whatever discussion that follows applies to any target of meditation. But the progress made in meditation is best if one takes *Pranava* as the target, for reasons that I discuss later. So, I refer to *Pranava*, as a typical object of meditation.

First stage of samādhi (*Vitarkānugata samādhi*)

In the previous section, we already discussed the first stage of *samādhi* namely *vitarkānugata samādhi*. As I said, this *samādhi* is attained due to total elimination of task unrelated thoughts. Whatever thoughts that still remain are about the object of meditation.

If we consider the case where *Pranava* is taken as the object of meditation, then during *Vitarkānugata samādhi* there would be thoughts about how the sound varies during the rising and decaying phases of the mantra, the way the air moves in and out of the lungs, and the meaning associated with *Pranava*.

Among these, the first two are about gross attributes of *Pranava* and the last is about the subtle aspects of *Pranava*. In addition, there would also be other thoughts that make one conscious of the act of meditation – that there is some object of meditation, there is a process called meditation, and finally that you are doing the meditation.

So, effectively, one is aware of gross attributes of the object of meditation, about its subtle attributes, about the act of meditation, and more importantly the experience of bliss due to complete lack of stress. This is the *Vitarkānugata samādhi*. The word *vitarka* stands for the thoughts related to gross things.

Second stage of samādhi (*Vicārānugata samādhi*)

As one continues to meditate, the thoughts related to the gross attributes of *Pranava* also gradually die down. Probably this happens because after sometime, the attention system does not find any novelty among the thoughts related to gross attributes and so it pays less and less attention to them. Grosser the attribute, lesser is the novelty in it, and so they get eliminated first. Novelty detection is one of the prominent features of our attention system. We always pay attention to something new rather than something that is already known.

Once thoughts related to gross attributes get eliminated, what we are left with are thoughts about subtle aspects of *Pranava*, thoughts about the act of meditation, and as always, the experience of bliss. This stage of *samādhi* is called *Vicārānugata samādhi*. The word *vicāra* stands for the thoughts related to subtle things.

Third stage of samādhi (*Ānandānugata samādhi*)

Further meditation eliminates even the thoughts about subtle attributes of *Pranava* owing to the same reason as that cited in the previous section. What we are left with is basically experience of bliss and the awareness about the act of meditation. There are no other thoughts whatsoever. Patanjali calls this stage as *Ānandānugata samādhi*. *Ānanda* or bliss is the dominant feature of this *samādhi* and hence the name.

Fourth stage of samādhi (*Asmitānugata samādhi*)

The awareness of bliss is also a thought – 'I experience bliss'. But even this thought dies down as one continues with the process of meditation. What are we left with in that stage? There is no longer any awareness of bliss. But there would be awareness about the act of meditation.

What does awareness of meditation mean? It means thoughts about the fact that there is an object of meditation, there is a process called meditation and finally there is someone who is meditating – or the awareness that 'I am meditating on *Pranava*'. This awareness about 'I am the one who meditates' or *Asmita* as it is called, is what gives the name *Asmitānugata samādhi* to this stage. In this stage, there are no thoughts about the object of meditation, no bliss, but only the awareness about self as involved in the act of meditation.

What happens when even this awareness goes?

It may look strange but even this stage would be reached if one continues to meditate beyond *Asmitānugata samādhi* explained in the previous section. Basically what happens is that even the thoughts about the existence of the object of meditation, existence of the process of meditation, and the existence of someone who is doing the meditation, as separate things, die down. It is as if the differentiation between the object, the act, and the actor has suddenly vanished.

This is the culminating stage of *samādhi* with awareness. In this stage there are no longer any thoughts, or any mental activity involved in perception or thinking. It is the final *Niruddha* – totally restrained - state of meditation. The mind is totally calm in this state.

What happens after this stage? That is what we will be seeing in the next chapter. Before I move on to that, let me briefly discuss two important questions.

How is *Pranava* specially suited as an object of meditation?

I said earlier that *Pranava* is considered to be the best object of meditation. The reasons could be many – some logically explainable and some based purely on faith. Let me look at explainable reasons.

Observe the gradual decay of sound in the trailing part of *Pranava* as shown in Figure 6.5. If you try listening to an audible *Pranava* sound, you will realize how more and more difficult it gets to listen to the sound as it gradually dies down. You need to pay more and more keen attention since the sound becomes less and less audible. More and more attention means greater involvement of the attention system. This could make the mind more and more engrossed and speed up the pace of progress in meditation.

Let me next take up one question that I had postponed during my discussion in Chapter 3, namely how devotional singing also can lead to the final stages of Yoga.

What happens in advanced stages of devotional singing?

Not all people who get involved in devotional singing will be able to reach the stages I am going to discuss in this section. But there are many reported cases where some advanced practitioners of devotional singing could get into the stages of *samādhi* which are normally experienced during the practice of Yoga. One well known example is that of Ramakrishna Paramahamsa (the Guru of Swami Vivekananda). He could easily get into *samādhi* while singing or even when listening to devotional songs.

After all, devotional singing is nothing but focusing the mind and body into the act of singing. In other words, the object of focus in devotional singing is the devotional songs.

As I discussed in Chapter 3, the right choice of devotional songs and associated mood of devotion eliminate thoughts relating to sense pleasures, ultimately leading to the *pratyāhāra* stage of Yoga.

As one progresses in singing, all thoughts except those related to the song vanish one by one, freeing the mind of all stress. Due to an outlet provided for emotions as well as due to the absence of conflicting thoughts, the person experiences bliss. This is something that happens to probably all the people who are seriously involved in devotional singing.

But what happens to advanced devotional singers is something more interesting. In the initial stages they remain aware of the lyrics of the song, the meaning of the words, the associated mood, the tune as well as the rhythm of the music.

But as one progresses further, gradually the focus on lyrics and meaning of the words vanishes and the person would be merely humming the tune with the associated mood. This is like the *Vicārānugata samādhi* of Yoga. He will be blissful, aware of the subtle aspects of the song (i.e. tune and rhythm) and also the act of singing.

Further down, he stops even the humming but remains blissful and aware of singing. This is the *Ānandānugata samādhi* stage of Yoga. This stage culminates in a stage where no experience remains and the person looses all awareness of not only the external world, but also the act of singing. This is like the final stage of *samādhi*.

Ramakrishna Paramahamsa gives a beautiful analogy to explain how this happens. He says that when a bee approaches a flower it initially makes lot of sound by fluttering its wings. It goes round and round the flower before it finally settles down on the petals and dips its suckers into the flower. It slowly draws in the nectar. It still keeps flapping its wings occasionally.

But once the nectar gets into its body, all the flapping stops; all the humming stops and there will be only the act of enjoying the nectar and nothing else! This is what happens when one gets completely engrossed in devotional singing – according to Ramakrishna Paramahamsa.

With these two pending issues sorted out, let us move on to the next chapter where I will discuss about what one 'experiences' in the final stage of *samādhi*. We will also see how this *samādhi* achieves what Patanjali aimed at, while putting forth his 8 step Yoga process.

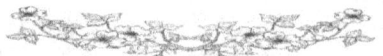

7 The vista beyond

In the previous chapter, we saw how the unruly ghost namely the mind can be shut off by the practice of prolonged meditation. In a step by step manner, the thoughts relating to sense perception, the thoughts unrelated to the object of the meditation, thoughts relating to the object of meditation, as well as those relating to the process of meditation itself, are stopped. Passing through a series of stages of *samādhi*, the mind appears to have finally stopped functioning. What next? What exists on the other side of this quietude? That is what we are going to discuss in this chapter.

The state beyond the mind

When I say 'state', I am not obviously talking about some state of the mind. I am just using this word for lack of any better word. I am using it to mean some reality that is beyond the reach of the mind. Ultimate state of *samādhi* is such a state that is beyond the domain of the mind. This state is the main topic discussed in ancient Upanishads (philosophic sections of the Vedas, ~ 2000 B.C.). You can have an overview of these Upanishads in my book "**Ancient Wisdom – Modern Viewpoints**",

The Upanishads assert that that state cannot be described by words, nor it can be logically inferred, it can neither be experienced in the way the sense objects are experienced. It is beyond the mind. An Upanishadic sage puts it as follows (*Kёna Upanishad* 1.3, 1.4)

> *The eyes cannot go there, nor the speech, not even the mind. We do not know, nor do we know of a way to explain it.*

It is surely different from whatever is known and it
is even beyond what is unknown (basically it is not
knowable by the mind) – this is what ancient
teachers told us.

What does one perceive in that state?

As we have already seen, during *samādhi*, sense perception is no long-er active. So, obviously, we cannot use the word 'perceive' in the way we use it to mean sense perception. So we need to assign different meaning to this word "perceive".

No matter what we mean by "perceive", the most difficult ques-tion to answer is – "who is the one who perceives, if anything!" We are so used to the word "we" that it is difficult to talk about any act without assuming that there is someone who is involved in the act. So we often take this "we" for granted.

However, the ancient Buddhists on the other hand, assert that there is none who actually "perceives" – neither during *samādhi* nor at any other time. For Buddhists "perceiving" is just a mechanical phe-nomenon without any sentient entity being behind the act. It is just a series of transformations that take place in the mind – a view similar to our current scientific view.

But Yoga, like its companion school Sänkhya and other related Vedic schools, firmly believes in the existence of a soul that is the sole beneficiary of actions performed by the mind. It asserts that it is the soul that uses the mind to interact with the world. Figure 7.1 shows how this soul sees an external object with the help of the senses and the mind, as a typical example.

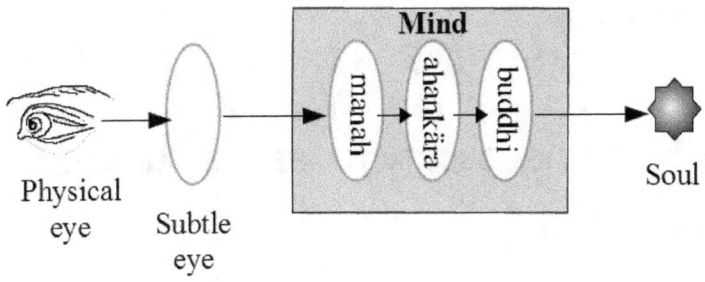

Figure 7.1 The way the soul sees external objects

This soul is the "we" we often keep referring to. The important question in that case is - what does this soul perceive when the mind has stopped functioning as a result of *samādhi?*

Even though most of the activities of the mind have stopped in that state, the way we moved towards the final stage of *samādhi* seems to indicate that the attention system of the mind is still functional. Let us assume that the soul normally perceives the external world, or the internally produced thoughts or dreams, using the attention system of the brain. Now, when there are no external inputs, nor any thoughts or dreams, what does the soul see through this attention system which is all the more sharply focused?

Patanjali (*Yoga Sutra* 1.3, 1.4) says that the soul sees itself!

At that time, the one who is seeing (i.e. the soul) remains established (i.e. assumes identity) with itself, as against the identity it had assumed based on the activities of the mind when the mind was active.

It is as if the soul is standing in front of a mirror! The mirror just reflects back whatever is in front of it. But when this mirror is transparent and when the soul can see through it – i.e. when the mind is active – the soul can no longer see itself. So it falsely assumes that it *is* what it sees – i.e. it assumes false identities, depending on its interactions with the world around.

I used this mirror analogy to explain what happens during final stage of *samādhi*, in my book **Psychology behind Yoga**. I will skip further details here.

Why is it necessary to realize our true identity?

The identity one normally assumes about oneself is based on one's interactions with the external world and based on what one thinks. We think we are a father, mother, son, daughter, teacher, businessman, politician, weak, powerful, intelligent, dumb, kind, cruel, and so on. Whatever we do is based on this assumed identity. We toil hard so that our wife and children can be taken care of. We grieve when our beloved are in difficulties. We feel bad when someone insults us.

An Upanishadic sage namely Yäjñavalkya sees the fallacy in our actions based on these assumed identities. He says that no one actually does anything for the sake of others – wife, children, and so on. All our actions are in the ultimate sense meant for our own benefit. That being the case, he asks - why not we first understand who we really are, and do something that benefits us eternally?

Why does our assumed identity not benefit us eternally? Why don't we enjoy various pleasures, comforts, wealth, and be happy? Yäjñavalkya gives two reasons why we cannot in the long run. He gives the following reasons.

1. Firstly, all pleasures, comforts and so on are experienced by our body. And we are not the body. Though it may appear that we are the real enjoyer, in the ultimate sense we are not.

2. Secondly, even if we assume that we enjoy all these pleasures, these pleasures cannot last long since all material things that give us these pleasures are perishable.

Here I am referring to the conversation between sage Yäjñavalkya and his wife Maitrëyi narrated in *Brahadäranyaka Upanishad*.

Apparently, once this sage decided to take up *sanyäsa* (renunciation). So he offered all his wealth to his wife. But his wife asked him whether this wealth could give her eternal peace. The answer Yäjñavalkya gave was interesting.

He first explained to her the illusory nature of our assumed identities. He also told her that knowing one's true identity is the only way one can get eternal peace. The worldly wealth can in no way give this peace. In Yäjñavalkya's opinion

One needs to ponder (i.e. meditate) over this 'self'
with full concentration. Once we understand who
this 'self' is, then we will know everything and that
will lead us to lasting peace.

No material wealth can give this lasting peace.
This is because all the material wealth is perishable
and temporary.

How is this 'true self' different from the identities we often assume? In another Upanishad namely the *Mändükya Upanishad* it is said that (part of *Mändükya Upanishad* verse 7)

Our true identity is most peaceful, most holy, all
encompassing, beyond time, and something worth
knowing.

Note the qualifiers 'peaceful', 'all encompassing', 'beyond time', 'worth knowing'. Let me elaborate on these words a bit.

- Peaceful: We are by nature peaceful. There is nothing extra we need to do to be peaceful. All that is needed is to throw away all false identities - source of our problems - that we have taken on ourselves and realize our true identity. And the peace is right there, as it always was.
- All encompassing: We often assume an identity that is circumscribed by our body. As compared to this, our true identity is limitless and all encompassing. This is the kind of experience one gets when one approaches the final stages of *samädhi*. One feels that all the restricted identities are getting dissolved into a limitless global identity. It is like a salt doll

that went to measure the depth of the sea – to quote the analogy given by Ramakrishna Paramahamsa in this regard. The doll just dissolves in the sea without retaining any separate identity.

- Beyond time: Our body has a beginning and an end. So also all the material entities as we see them. But our true identity has neither beginning nor an end. It is timeless. It always existed and would continue to exist forever, no matter what happens to the body. This is the firm belief of the Upanishads.

- Worth knowing: It is worth knowing because the cause of our miseries is our forgetting our true nature. Once we know who we really are, then there is no misery, no suffering whatsoever.

This is what the Upanishad is saying. As compared to this true identity, our assumed identities have several limitations and are rarely peaceful.

Now the important question that arises is - why don't we just assume our true identity that is limitless? The Upanishad says that it is not sufficient to know that we have a true identity that is limitless. We have to 'realize' it through a proper process (part of *Mändükya Upanishad* verse 7).

It (i.e. the true identity) cannot be known through the senses. It cannot be explained the way we explain an object that can be perceived through our senses. It can neither be inferred, nor is it within the reach of our thoughts. It has no attributes using which it can be known. It is something that has to be realized.

And the way to realize it is through meditation. If you recall the comments of Gaudapäda (on *Mändükya Upanishad*) that we discussed in **Part II** of this book series, even Gaudapäda says that

*With the help of proper process one should bring
the mind - which is normally dispersed amidst objects of desire and enjoyment - under discipline.*

*When the mind does not become lost (as in the deep
sleep state), nor is scattered (as in the wakeful or
dreaming/ideating states) but is motionless (as in
samādhi state) it realizes as well as becomes the ultimate reality.*

Having said that our true identity is most peaceful how is it that
our assumed identities force us to go through miseries? In what way
the practice of Yoga can take us out of this suffering? These are
questions that become predominant for anyone who wants to enjoy
eternal peace.

How does Yoga bring about lasting peace?

Before we can understand this, let us first know why we undergo
suffering in spite of the fact that we are inherently peaceful.

Due to various assumed identities, we tend to act in such a way
that these actions ultimately lead us to suffering. Why does a soul that
is peaceful by nature and the one that is inherently holy, indulge in
such actions fully knowing the consequences? What motivates us to
do such things?

Yoga says that the preset impressions (*Klesha*) in our minds motivate us. Under the influence of these impressions we perform various actions that ultimately lead us into suffering. These preset impressions are the spiritual counterparts of genetic imprints. They are
like the preset programs that run our body/mind combination. They
come with us right from birth. Even the ancient Buddhists who

didn't accept the concept of soul assumed the existence of such pre-set impressions.

During our lifetime, we indulge in various actions motivated by these preset impressions. Each of our actions leaves back its own indelible impression that further fortifies the already existing impressions. And the accumulation of these impressions goes on, making them stronger over a period of time, unless checked. We will see in the next section how this can be checked. Before that, let us look at these preset impressions a bit more in detail.

The five preset impressions (*Klesha*)

Patanjali lists (*Yoga Sutra* 2.3) the following as the five preset impressions that not only motivate us to completely get engrossed in the world, but also get us into many problems.

> *Wrong knowledge (Avidya), wrong association (Asmita), craving for pleasure (Räga), aversion to suffering (Dvesha) and innate desire to exist (Abhinivesa) are the five preset impressions (Klesha).*

Let us see what these five preset impressions are, one by one.

1. Wrong understanding (*Avidya*)

As per Patanjali, the wrong understanding has the following aspects.

- Mistaking transient things as permanent. Our lives are transient and have a definite end. But still we assume that it is permanent and indulge in activities that ultimately result in suffering. We amass wealth and in the process hurt others. We indulge in hatred and violence, totally forgetting that we too are vulnerable to them and whatever wealth we have amassed is not going to last long.

- <u>Seeing beauty in ugly things.</u> We get attracted to physical beauty and tend to crave for sense pleasures. We forget the maxim "beauty is only skin deep". Underneath lie all dirty things but we ignore all that.
- <u>Mistaking suffering as pleasure.</u> All sense pleasures are associated with three fold consequences –
  - o they have adverse aftereffects
  - o they induce craving for more pleasure, and
  - o they leave back indelible impressions on our mind.

Viewed from this point of view, Patanjali says that all sense pleasures are nothing but suffering.
- <u>Mistaking the body for the soul.</u> Yoga believes that "we" are not the body, but the soul. But we often forget this and assume that we are identical with our body.

Patanjali says that this wrong understanding is the mother of rest of the four preset impressions. In other words, the other impressions are born due to this wrong understanding. Let us look at rest of the four preset impressions.

2. Wrong association (*Asmita*)

We often hold ourselves to be the one who performs any action. But Yoga sees these actions as performed by our body and says that we wrongly arrogate the consequences of these actions on ourselves. As a result, we suffer. When we do something, say when we eat something

- there is an object that is eaten
- there is an act of eating
- there is a body/mind that is involved in this act
- there is "we" who enjoys from this act of eating.

But we generally assume that it is "we" who eats as well as enjoys from eating. As per Yoga, this is a wrong association. Yoga calls this wrong association as *Asmita*. It says that "we" don't eat but the body does. So the consequent enjoyment or suffering does not strictly belong to us. This applies to any other sense pleasure we undergo. Yoga says that this wrong association leads to suffering.

The companion school of Yoga namely the *Sänkhya* asserts that this wrong association is the root cause of all our suffering. You can find how Sänkhya argues its point in **Part II** of this series.

3. Craving (*Räga*)

When we experience some sense enjoyment, our mind remembers this enjoyment. Later on, whenever our mind remembers this pleasant experience it desires to have it again. Repeated enjoyment creates insatiable urge to have it again and again. Further it leads to greed, preventing anyone from having it. Yoga calls this impression as craving or *Räga*.

4. Aversion to suffering (*Dvesha*)

When we undergo an unpleasant experience, our mind remembers that too. This results in aversion to the object that created this unpleasant experience, anger towards the persons responsible for the experience and finally hatred. This is called *Dvesha*.

5. Innate desire to exist (*Abhinivesa*)

All living beings have an innate desire to continue to exist. This is what motivates us to do everything – in order to continue to exist. No one wants to die. This strong desire to exist is called *Abhinivesa*.

According to Yoga, these 5 preset impressions are the ones that motivate us not only to exist and perform actions, but also the ones that lead to our suffering. These are so strong that one cannot easily escape from them.

Patanjali says (*Yoga Sutra 2.2*) that Yoga can reduce this overpowering influence of these preset impressions.

> *The Yoga practice is meant for getting into the*
> *samādhi stage as well as for minimizing the effects*
> *of preset impressions.*

How does Yoga minimize the effect of these preset impressions that seem to be impossible to overcome? That is what we will be seeing next.

How does Yoga minimize the overpowering influence of Kleshas?

Patanjali says that when one remains in *samādhi* stage, new impressions get formed in the mind. And these new impressions gradually nullify the preset impressions. (*Yoga Sutra* 1.50, 1.51)

> *The impressions that get formed when one is in*
> *samādhi nullify other (preset) impressions.*

> *When all impressions get nullified, the person*
> *reaches a seedless (nirbīja) state of samādhi.*

So, over a period of time these preset impressions are made ineffective like the burnt seeds. Burnt seeds can't germinate. Patanjali says that these preset impressions become ineffective by prolonged practice of Yoga. No preset impressions, means no associated suffering.

Patanjali uses the specific word 'seed' (*bīja*) to suggest that the preset impressions are like the seeds that germinate to produce rebirth which is when the whole process starts all over again. When these seeds are burnt and made ineffective, there can be no more births and the suffering ends. This idea rests on the belief that cycle of births and rebirths is something that breeds suffering.

Cycle of births and rebirths as the perpetual breeding ground of all suffering

Rebirth is a strongly ingrained belief in most ancient religions. Not only the ancient Greeks, but also Vedic Indians as well as Buddhists believed in rebirth. It is said that even ancient Judaism believed in this concept though its later offshoots don't seem to have faith in it.

In **Part II** we saw how even some of the modern scientists assert that rebirth is not just a belief but scientifically verifiable reality. They offer volumes of recorded 'real life incidents' which according to them support the possibility of rebirth beyond doubt.

Surprisingly, the Vedic Indians who firmly believed in the existence of a soul that goes through the apparently endless cycle of births and rebirths, as well as the Buddhists who didn't even accept the concept of soul, both believed in rebirth! Each had an elaborate theory about how it happens. Not so amazingly, their theories had lot in common. I have discussed the process of rebirth as per both these schools in **Part II** of this book series.

Ancient philosophers considered cycle of births, deaths, and rebirths as the breeding ground of all our suffering. These rebirths are supposed to be driven by the preset impressions as well as the impressions left back by the actions that we perform during our life time. These combined impressions are called *Karma* by the Vedic group and *Kamma* by the Buddhists. Both these groups have elaborate theories on how these impressions buildup during our lifetime.

While impressions left behind by *Samādhi* makes preset impressions ineffective, the Yoga practice itself prevents new accumulations of the *Karma*. Together they gradually release one from the cycle of births and rebirths. That is the ultimate deliverance, a deliverance from all miseries.

Some points to ponder about

Throughout this book I have tried to explain various Yoga processes in scientific terms. That would make our understanding more objec-

tive and prevent us from falling trap to wrong conceptions.
Ideally one would like to bring the entire Yoga system into the ambit of scientific investigation, to the extent possible. That would require understanding of the working of Yoga in objective terms.

However, the final state of *samādhi*, what one experiences in that state, and the after effects of that state are generally considered to be beyond objective verification. Most people believe that these are very subjective things that can never be objectively studied. In this context, there are two important questions that are worth pondering about.

1. Firstly, in what way *samādhi* is different from deep sleep?
2. Secondly, are the impressions supposedly left behind by the *samādhi* on the mind (after effects of *samādhi*) verifiable?

Let us take up these two questions one by one.

1. In what way *samadhi* is different from deep sleep?

Superficially, it may appear that there is not much of difference between deep sleep and *samādhi*. In deep sleep as well as in *samādhi*, sense perception is inhibited, so also the thoughts and dreams. That being the case, what really differentiates *samādhi* from deep sleep?

Interestingly the *Māndūkya Upanishad* seems to highlight this difference. I have discussed in greater detail about this Upanishad in **Part II** of this book series. This Upanishad specifically deals with different states of our existence. Basically, this Upanishad talks about 4 states of our existence, namely

1. wakeful (*Jāgrta*) state
2. dreaming (*Swapna*) state
3. deep sleep (*Sushupti*) state
4. something beyond these three states (i.e. *Turīya*)

The *Māndūkya Upanishad* defines deep sleep state as follows (*Māndūkya Upanishad* 5)

> *Deep sleep (Sushupti) is a state in which one does*
> *not desire any sense objects (i.e. does not engage in*
> *sense perception), nor does he dream. It is as if his*
> *consciousness is frozen. But he is in deep state of*
> *bliss and this state (i.e. state of deep sleep) is a ga-*
> *teway to either the wakeful state or the dreaming*
> *state (i.e. one can either wakeup from this deep*
> *sleep state or once again enter into a dreaming*
> *state).*

Upanishad calls the ultimate stage of *samādhi* as *Turïya* state. The Upanishad differentiates this ultimate state from deep sleep state as follows (part of *Māndūkya Upanishad* verse 7)

> *In that state (i.e. the Turïya state), one's attention*
> *is not directed to external world, nor is it directed*
> *to the inner dream world (probably that includes*
> *thoughts). At the same time, it is not as if one's*
> *consciousness is frozen (unlike the deep sleep state).*
> *Also, it cannot be said that one is not aware of an-*
> *ything. In fact, one becomes omniscient in this state.*

So the difference lies in the fact that in one case – i.e. deep sleep state– the consciousness is inactive (frozen) and in the other case – i.e. *samādhi* state – the consciousness is highly active though it does not attend to anything external or internal.

In **Part I** of this book series, we saw how the philosophical concept of consciousness can be viewed in terms of the functioning of the brain where the attention system coordinates the diverse activities of the brain to arrive at a single coherent percept, which we normally define as conscious experience.

Translating the above assertions of the Upanishad into neurological terms, probably we can conclude as follows.

When we are in a deep state of sleep, our attention system is almost shutoff (frozen). That is the reason why we perceive neither the external inputs, nor the thoughts or the dreams that are internally generated.

Now recollect the way our attention system progresses during continued meditation, as we discussed in Chapter 6. Though the attention system neither attends to external events nor the internal events, we see it becoming more and more active and focused sharper. That means it is still capable of attending. This almost matches the description given by the Upanishad.

So, probably, during the deep state of meditation, neural structures corresponding to the attention system get highly active, while most of the other activities of the brain including the so called 'idle mode activities' may be shutdown.

It is generally reported that even the breathing as well as heart rates drop as one progresses into advanced meditative states. Traditionally, it is said that when one enters *samädhi*, one's breathing stops. Actually, the breathing may not stop but probably becomes feeble. That means that even the autonomous nervous systems show a drastic dip in their activity.

If these assertions are valid, then these measurable effects of deep states of meditation can be verified scientifically using fMRI and such other means.

2. Are the after effects of *samädhi* verifiable?

In the previous question, we talked about what probably happens – in neurological terms – during *samädhi*. It is also interesting to probe whether there are any measurable aftereffects of *samädhi*.

We have no idea whether the impressions left behind by *samädhi* as talked about by Patanjali have any corresponding effects on the physical brain. Assuming that the preset impressions that we talked about earlier and their weakening due to the impressions caused by the *samädhi*, have some corresponding neural correlates , we must be able to observe some structural changes in the brain, due to prolonged practice of Yoga.. If this is possible, we can bring even the after effects of *samädhi* within the purview of scientific validation.

The subjective experience of *samädhi* may escape scientific validation and remain forever illusive, though.

Not all of the intense and quite involved processes of Yoga that we discussed in the foregoing chapters may be practicable by all. Probably, only highly motivated people can reach till the end of the entire process of Yoga. But that does not prevent others from taking advantage of Yoga. In the next chapter I suggest some simple and quick assortment of Yoga processes for such people.

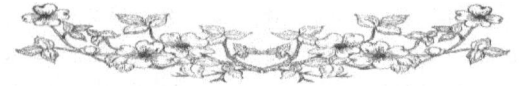

8 A 30 minutes Yoga for everyone

In today's superfast life style, most people may find it hard to devote sufficient time for Yoga. Also, not all people may be interested in achieving the ultimate states of Yoga. But physical and mental health, freedom from stress, and capability to perform well in one's chosen profession is something that everyone would like to achieve.

Considering the fact that Yoga helps in achieving these goals, it is advisable to devote at least half hour each day for Yoga, and reap its benefits. More than the duration of practice, what is important is the regularity and sincerity.

For those of you who have hectic weekdays, I have split the practice in to two categories – *weekday practice* and *weekend practice*. Each of these need half hour of time and I am sure you would see positive results in a matter of one month of practice. None of these practices need anything more than your time and devotion. So do try them.

All the required information is given in the preceding chapters. So I will not repeat those details. Refer to the chapters as indicated below. Before starting the regular practice regime, get yourselves familiar with various Yoga processes – whether it is different Yoga postures, mind focusing techniques or the meditation techniques. Start the actual schedule only after you are comfortable with the chosen processes.

Weekday practice

The recipe I have chosen for weekday practice is a good mix of sharpening focusing skills, developing a calm and stress free mind, as well as remaining healthy.

The first two should prepare you for the hectic day ahead. They are preferably done early in the morning and most importantly – the same time each day.

The last one namely the processes to remain healthy can be performed in the evening at some convenient time. Let me now explain each of these components – the morning routine as well as the evening routine.

Weekday morning practice (20 minutes)

Early morning hours are beneficial to the practice of mind oriented Yoga processes in more than one way. It is the most peaceful time of the day. The mind and the body would be fresh after a good night sleep and there would be fewer distractions.

Start the practice preferably after bath to feel fresh and alert. Don't indulge in any vigorous activity just before the practice. Also, keeping silent for sometime before the practice, helps in keeping the mind amenable to modulation.

First 10 minutes

For 10 minutes, practice any one of the techniques described in Chapter 5 to sharpen your focusing skills. You can do the controlled breathing, or the mindful-breathing, or the candle gazing technique. I would recommend mantra chanting for the next step.

This step not only helps in sharpening your mental focus but also prepares you for the next step since it calms the mind and frees it from distractions.

Next 10 minutes

For the next 10 minutes do the meditation as described in Chapter 6, choosing any of the objects of focus as discussed in that chapter.

You can mediate on the image of your favorite deity, or some religious symbol, a burning flame, some sound, and so on. For best results, I would recommend meditating on the *Pranava* sound as I discussed in that chapter. Meditating on the *Pranava* sound would help calming the mind quickly and make you stress free.

However, most of us would like to strike a balance between calmness of the mind and ability to perform multi-tasking. I am not suggesting that meditating on the *Pranava* sound would inevitably make you less capable of multi-tasking. A short 10 minutes practice should not have any such effect, though prolonged duration – say hours – of meditation on *Pranava* has the potential to calm the mind so much that you may find it difficult to do multi-tasking. So, the best alternative for most people is to do mantra chanting for 10 minutes rather than meditating on *Pranava*.

As I discussed in Chapters 5 and 6, the specific mantra I had talked about for this purpose has the potential to both calm the mind, and at the same time keep it agile enough to allow you to do multi-tasking. I have given more details of this mantra as well as various alternate ways of using it, in my book "**A mantra to enhance your mental capabilities**". I have also provided sound clippings of this mantra in my blog **http://doctor-king-online.blogspot.com**. Please make use of them.

Evening practice (10 minutes)

Do the *Sun salutation* described in 4. A 10 minute practice of *Sun salutation* alone may be a bit tiring in the beginning. You can club it with the *all limbs posture*, also discussed in the same chapter, if you prefer. Both these practices have the advantage of body exercise as well as controlled breathing. This should not only improve your physical health, but also make you stress free and focused.

Weekend practice

I have a slightly different emphasis for the weekend practice. I recommend that you do this practice in the evenings. This practice is more focused on the body and emotional wellbeing.

First 10 minutes

This part is same as that explained for the week day evening practice.

Next 20 Minutes

For the next 20 minutes, I would recommend devotional singing – either solo or in a group. In either case, take care to follow the instructions given in Chapter 3. Avoid pomp and show. Don't convert it into a mechanical ritual, but make it a purposeful act.

Even if you are not a religiously minded person, for the reasons I stated in Chapter 3 and in Chapter 6, devotional singing has several positive benefits irrespective of your faith. The benefits discussed in these chapters are independent of the existence or otherwise of God. So you can make use of this technique to your advantage. It is needless to stress that this practice would not clash with your religious orientation.

This devotional singing not only gives you spiritual peace, but also provides an outlet for your emotions, gives you freedom from stress, and most importantly an opportunity to mingle with your dear ones.

Combined practice

For those of you who can squeeze in more time, I would recommend doing both weekday as well as weekend practices each day of the week, weekday morning practices in the morning and weekend practices in the evening of the same day. That would give you all round benefit. Try to find time to the extent possible. You will be greatly rewarded.

General life style

As I said in Chapter 2, the root cause of most of our problems and stress is the wrong style of our living. We need to shift from an individual centered life style to a more all encompassing life style. We need to act as per the *Dharma* as I discussed in that chapter. This does not mean that you have to follow some new religion. All religions have this *Dharma* at their base. So try to practice it to the extent possible.

Be honest, be kind to everyone, be content with what you have, keep the luxuries to the minimum, remain calm, cultivate positive attitude to life, and so on. This not only makes you a good individual, but also a healthy, stress free individual who can perform his tasks to the best of his abilities and achieve success in life.

Continue to follow your chosen religion, giving more emphasis to its core values rather than to the mechanical rituals.

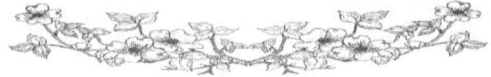

Epilogue

When I started this 3 part series, namely the *Marvels of the Mind*, what I had uppermost in my mind was to finally explain the apparently mysterious practice like Yoga in scientific terms. More than just an intellectual pursuit, what I had in my mind was to clear lot of misconceptions, so that the full potential of this marvelous system, that was developed thousands of years ago, is realized.

I built the foundation in **Part I** by discussing our scientific advancement in the effort to understand mind – the most marvelous entity. This is a highly specialized subject. But I have tried to explain it in simple terms so that its prominent contributions can be utilized in understanding Yoga better.

In **Part II** , I took you through an altogether different journey – a journey through almost 2000 years of philosophic attempts to understand the mind and beyond. This is a very interesting subject in itself. But it also introduced the reader to some of the concepts that are essential in understanding the metaphysical aspects of Yoga.

In this third part, I kept our current scientific advances in the background, while explaining this thousands of year old practice namely Yoga. Yoga is a subject that spans science, philosophy as well as spirituality. The exposure I had provided in Part I and Part II comes handy in understanding all these aspects of Yoga.

For more practically oriented people, I have also made this book a sort of manual or guide for the practice of Yoga. If one chooses to, one can skip scientific and logical explanations provided about the working of Yoga, and limit oneself to only its practical aspects. However, I will advise you not to take that option. You stand to gain a lot if you understand the theory behind Yoga before you seriously undertake its practice.

Best of luck! Start with your journey through Yoga practice, fully armed with all that you need to know.

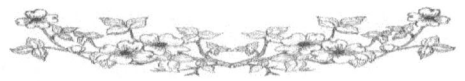

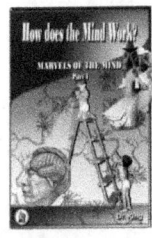

Thank you for reading my book. I hope you enjoyed reading it. Please give me your feedback through book reviews. I appreciate that very much. You may contact me through my blog at http://doctor-king-online.blogspot.com I will be happy to hear from you. If you have any specific questions or suggestions, indicate them through my blog and I will surely respond to them.

You may also be interested in reading my other books available through several online vendors.

My recent Books

Following is the list of my recent books. Some of these books are now available from one or more of online bookstores such as

Amazon, Scribd, Smashwords, Apple iBookstores, Barnes & Noble, Sony, Kobo, Flipkart Diesel eBook Store, eBooks Eros, Baker & Taylor, Page Foundry ,WH Smith in the UK, FNAC in France and Portugul, Livraria Cultura in Brazil, Angus & Robertson in Australia, Bookworld in Australia, Indigo in Canada, Collins in Australia, Feltrinelli in Italy, Libris in the Netherlands, Paper Plus in New Zealand, Play in Great Britain, Rakuten in Japan, Rakuten in the US, Whitcoulls in New Zealand.

Please look for them in your favorite book store. You can always use the book title in your search to see if the book is available in your favorite bookstore. I have given the appropriate links for your convenience in my blog http://doctor-king-online.blogspot.com

How does the Mind work? (Marvels of the mind Part I)

Book synopsis: The mind is probably the most complex of the nature's creations. It is an extremely fascinating and intriguing entity, probably beyond the reach of human beings to have a complete understanding.

This is the first part of a 3 part series namely *Marvels of the Mind,* discussing various aspects of the mind. While the second and third parts of this series cover philosophic and spiritual facets of the mind, this part focuses mainly on the current scientific views about how the mind functions.

While several books that explain various aspects of this wonderful subject do exist, the subject is too specialized and beyond the grasp of general readers. The technical jargon used in these books needs proper background. Besides, books often don't give up-to-date information that can only be found in research journals and conference proceedings.

Most readers may neither have access to these books or journals, nor have the necessary background to follow intense technical literature. The current book tries to overcome some of these problems by explaining this subject in an easy to understand style with lot of simple day-to-day examples. The book follows a structured approach to cater for the needs of readers with varying backgrounds and interests. The reader can pick and choose the detail depending on the interest and aptitude.

Apart from providing the readers with the latest scientific information about the functioning of the mind, the book lays the foundation for the discussion in later parts of this series about the working of Yoga and Meditation.

Important missing dimensions in our current understanding of the Mind (Marvels of the mind Part II)

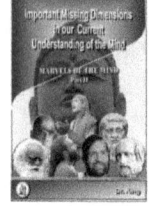 Book synopsis: Our current scientific achievements in understanding the working of the mind are commendable. However, in it's over insistence on objectivity science seems to have overlooked some important dimensions of the mind. There are many questions science fails to provide satisfactory answer.

Interestingly, many of these questions were addressed by ancient philosophies and probably in the true scientific spirit we should look at these philosophies with an open mind.

This second part of the 3 part series **Marvels of the Mind** focuses on these missed dimensions and how ancient philosophies address them. A range of ancient philosophies, amazingly well conceptualized, that look at different aspects of the mind are discussed in the current book.

There is the ancient philosophy of Plato who points out the limitations of our sense perception, the elaborate psychology of ancient

Buddhists that almost parallels with our scientific understanding, the philosophy of Šankara who even questions the reality of existence and the concept of domains beyond mind that are the focus of ancient Upanishads. All these, and more, are explained clearly in this second part of the series.

These philosophies compel us to rethink on our current definition of science and its approach. The book also provides a smooth transition point from science to philosophy and finally to domains beyond both these.

How and Why of Yoga and Meditation (Marvels of the mind Part III)

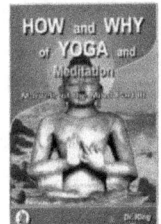

Book synopsis: This book gives a clear insight into various aspects of Yoga, while providing scientifically backed explanation about how various Yoga processes achieve their intended purposes and why they are designed that way. Such clarity is needed to understand Yoga in a more scientific manner and to realize its full potential.

The book also explains in a step by step manner how various processes of Yoga, namely the body postures, breathing techniques and meditation are performed and why each of these processes is essential to attain complete benefit of Yoga.

This book is a good guide for anyone who wants to practice Yoga.

Yöga Facts: *Answers to some important questions about Yöga*

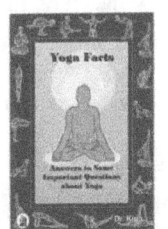

Book synopsis: Going by the large number of books on Yoga that are published and sold both through printed as well as electronic media, this ancient science seems to be very popular. While various things are propagated in the name of Yoga, there is often mismatch between expectations and achievements.

This short set of questions and answers clears some of the misconceptions about Yoga by drawing attention to the original works on Yoga dating back more than 2000 years. Questions that often arise as a result of commercially motivated propaganda are answered in a matter of fact manner. At the same time, this book reassures a sincere Yoga practitioner, that the goal is not only achievable but worth the effort.

Some of the questions discussed include - controversies due to adverse scientific findings about Yoga, why many people fail to achieve any progress in spite of sincere efforts, and so on.

Psychology behind Yoga: *Lesser known insights into the ancient science of Yoga*

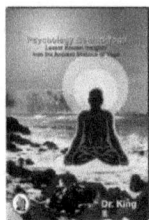

Book synopsis: Though Yöga is well known as a process to achieve the ultimate realization, not much attention is paid to its psychological underpinnings. This book builds up the theory behind Yoga based on descriptions given in ancient texts such as Yoga sutra of Patanjali (~200 B.C.) and Sänkhya Kärika of Isvara Krshna (~300 A.D.). This understanding is essential to get a complete grasp of the Yöga process.

This book clearly explains the concept of mind as defined in Yoga Sutra and Sänkhya Kärika, various states this mind can be in, and how by a step by step process the mind can be nudged into the ultimate desirable state namely the Samadhi. It discusses various hindrances one encounters while going through this process as well as how these can be overcome. As often mistaken, samädhi is not a single state but a series of progressive states one goes through as one progresses into the Yoga practice. This book explains those stages both with reference to the original sources as well as through simple analogies.

The ultimate state of Yoga, namely the niruddha state of mind is also very well explained, its implications and what exactly happens in that stage.

Ancient wisdom – Modern viewpoints: *Interesting picks from ancient Indian scriptures*

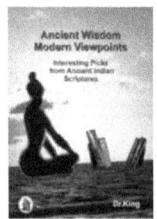

Book synopsis: This book captures the essence of ancient Indian scriptures, analyzing them from today's point of view. The scriptures selected are mainly the eleven Upanishads (parts of Vedic literature), Bhagavad Geetha (most important book of Indian philosophy) and the Manu Smrthi (one of the most ancient law books by Manu). All these scriptures were composed more than 2500 years ago and influence the Indian way of life even to this day. In addition to these primary scriptures, this book also cross references several other ancient Indian scriptures such as Yoga Sutra of Patanjali, Sänkhya Kärika, Närada Bhakti sutra, and Dammapada.

Some of the key aspects of each of these three main scriptures – Upanishads, Bhagavad Geetha and Manu Smrthi - are picked and presented in 6 short, crisp articles. While writing these articles, the original Sanskrit texts are relied upon with minimal re-interpretation. Adequate references to the original Sanskrit verses are given in most places, to impart authenticity to the rendering. To help the readers who may not be familiar with Sanskrit, simple English translations of these verses are also provided.

This is an ideal book for anyone who wants to have a quick overview of most of the ancient Indian scriptures. The book gives a wealth of information and surely a key to the treasure of ancient Indian scriptures.

Around the Mind

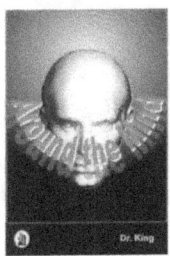

Book synopsis: Mind may probably be the most intriguing thing that has fascinated human beings, philosophers as well as the scientists, for thousands of years. This book summarizes our current scientific views on the Mind, the questions that arise due to that view, the efforts by ancient philosophies to address these questions and probably a possibility of going beyond the realms of current scientific approach.

A Mantra to enhance your mental capabilities

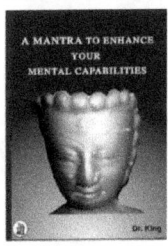

Book synopsis: For thousands of years, millions of people have taken advantage of one mantra which is believed to enhance the mental capabilities. Though it is used even today, it has become a prerogative of a small minority of people and seems to be going into the oblivion. The ravages of time has seriously rendered this potent mantra into an article of religious faith and deep rooted superstition, depriving the vast majority from realizing its benefits.

This book opens up this mantra to all those who are desirous of enhancing their mental capabilities. It discusses various aspects of this mantra and explains in a step by step fashion how anyone can take advantage of this mantra.

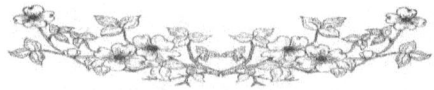

Bibliography

1. **Bhadanta Anuruddhäcäriya.** *Abhidhammattha Sangaha.*
2. **Buddhist Monks.** *Tipitaka - the Pali canon.* ~ 300 B.C. Recordings of Buddhas teachings by his disciples.
3. *Gheranda Samhita.*
4. **Patanjali.** *Yoga Sutra.* ~200 B.C.
5. *Siva Samhita.*
6. **Ïšvara Kršhna.** *Sänkhya Kärika.* ~ 3rd century A.D.
7. *Mändükya Upanishad.* ~2000 B.C.
8. **Gaudapäda.** *Mändükya Kärika.* ~ 6th century A.D.
9. **Vyäsa.** *Bhagavad Geetha (as part of Epic Mahäbhärata).* ~ 300 B.C.
10. **Nàrada Mahà Thera.** *A Manual of Abhidhamma.* s.l. : Publication of the Buddhist Missionary Society.
11. **John T. Bullitt (Editor).** *Tipitaka: The Pali Canon.* s.l. : Access to Insight, http://www.accesstoinsight.org/tipitaka/index.html.
12. **Swämi Virupäkshänanda.** *Sänkhya Kärika of Ïšvara Kršhna with The Tattva Kaumudi of Sri Väcaspati Misra.* s.l. : Sri Rämakrishna Math, Madras.
13. **Swämi Ädidevänada.** *Pätanjala Yöga Darshana with Vyäsa Bhäshya.* s.l. : Sri Rämakrishna Äshrama, Mysore.
14. **Swami Gambhiränada.** *Eight Upanishads Part II .* s.l. : Advaita Äshrama Calcutta.
15. **Swämi Ädidevänada.** *Mändükya Upanishad and Gaudapäda Kärika.* s.l. : Sri Rämakrishna Äshrama, Mysore.
16. **Swämi Somanäthänanda.** *Upanishad Bhävadhäre.* s.l. : Sri Rämakrishna Äshrama, Mysore.
17. **Swami Gambhiränada.** *Bhagavad Gïta with commentary of Šankaräcärya.* s.l. : Advaita Äshrama Calcutta.
18. **Swämi Ädidevänada.** *Srimadbhagavadgita.* s.l. : Sri Rämakrishna Äshrama, Mysore.
19. **Swami Svätmaräma .** *Hatayoga Pradeepika.* ~15th century A.D.
20. *EFFECT OF YOGA EXERCISES ON ACHIEVEMENT,MEMORY AND REASONING ABILITY.* **Nilesh Gajjar.** 1, December 2012, International Journal for Research

in Education (IJRE), Vol. 1.

21. *Effect of Yoga on Arrhythmia Burden, Anxiety, Depression, and Quality of Life in Paroxysmal Atrial Fibrillation.* **Dhanunjaya Lakkireddy, et.al.** 11, 2013, Journal of the American College of Cardiology, Vol. 61.

22. *THE BENEFITS OF YOGA: A BRIEF SUMMARY OF EVIDENCE-BASED YOGA RESEARCH.* **Deborah Roberts.** April 2013, Yoga Australia.

23. *The Health Benefits of Yoga and Exercise: A Review of Comparison Studies.* **Alyson Ross, et.al.** 1, 2010, THE JOURNAL OF ALTERNATIVE AND COMPLEMENTARY MEDICINE, Vol. 16.

24. *Yoga for Arthritis: A Scoping Review.* **Steffany Haaz, et.al.** 1, February 2011, Rheum Dis Clin North Am., Vol. 37.

25. *Yoga for Persistent Pain: New Findings and Directions for an Ancient Practice.* **Anava A. Wren, et.al.** 3, March 2011, Pain. 2011, Vol. 152.

26. *Yoga clinical research review.* **Tiffany Field.** 2011, Complementary Therapies in Clinical Practice.

27. *Efficacy of Yoga: Cognitive and Human Relationship Training for Correcting Maladjustment Behaviour in Deviant School Boys.* **R. Kannappan, et.al.** April 2008, Journal of the Indian Academy of Applied Psychology, Vol. 34.

28. *Evaluation of the Effectiveness and Efficacy of Iyengar Yoga Therapy on Chronic Low Back Pain.* **Kimberly Williams, et.al.** 19, 2009, SPINE, Vol. 34.

29. *Feasibility and acceptability of yoga for treatment of hot flushes: A pilot trial.* **Beth E. Cohen, et.al.** 2006, Maturitas.

30. *The efficacy of a comprehensive lifestyle modification programme based on yoga in the management of bronchial asthma: a randomized controlled trial.* **Ramaprabhu Vempati, et.al.** 9, July 2009, BMC Pulmonary Medicine, Vol. 37.

31. *Yoga for Cancer Patients and Survivors.* **Julienne E. Bower, et.al.** 3, July 2005, Julienne E. Bower,, Vol. 12.

32. *Yoga Therapy Decreases Dyspnea-Related Distress and Improves Functional Performance in People with Chronic Obstructive Pulmonary Disease: A Pilot Study.* **DorAnne Donesky-Cuenco, et.al.** 3, 2009, THE JOURNAL OF ALTERNATIVE AND COMPLEMENTARY MEDICINE, Vol. 15.

33. *A Pilot Study of a Yoga and Meditation Intervention for Dementia Caregiver Stress.* **Lynn C. Waelde, et.al.** 6, 2004, JOURNAL OF CLINICAL PSYCHOLOGY, Vol. 60.

34. *Treatment of Chronic Insomnia with Yoga: A Preliminary Study with Sleep–Wake Diaries.* **Sat Bir S. Khalsa.** 4, 2004, Applied Psychophysiology and Biofeedback, Vol. 29.

35. *Yoga in cardiac health (A Review).* **Satyajit R. Jayasinghe.** 2004, European Journal of Cardiovascular Prevention and Rehabilitation, Vol. 11.

36. *Yoga for bronchial asthma: a controlled study.* **R NAGARATHNA, H R NAGENDRA.** 1985, BRITISH MEDICAL JOURNAL, Vol. 291.

37. **S.N.Omkar.** *Student Upliftment & Rejuvenation through YogA.* s.l. : Yoga Mandir, 2007.

38. *Brain Facts : A PRIMER ON THE BRAIN AND NERVOUS SYSTEM.* s.l. : Society for Neuroscience, 2008.

39. *Cooperation between the default mode network and the frontal–parietal network in the production of an internal train of thought.* **Jonathan Smallwood, et.al.** 2012, Brain Research.

40. *Emerging concepts for the dynamical organization of resting-state activity in the brain.* **Gustavo Deco, et.al.** 2011, Neuroscience, Vol. 12.

41. *Momentary Interruptions Can Derail the Train of Thought.* **Erik M. Altmann, et.al.** 1, 2014, Journal of Experimental Psychology, Vol. 143.

42. *The Persistence of Thought: Evidence for a Role of Working Memory in the Maintenance of Task-Unrelated Thinking.* **Daniel B. Levinson, et.al.** 4, April 2012, Psychol Sci., Vol. 23.

43. *Wandering Minds: The Default Network and Stimulus-Independent thought.* **Malia F. Mason, et.al.** 2007, Science.

44. *Medial prefrontal cortex and self-referential mental Medial prefrontal cortex and self-referential mental brain function.* **Debra A. Gusnard, et.al.** 7, March 2001, PNAS, Vol. 98.

45. *Depression, Stress, and Anhedonia: Toward a Synthesis and Integrated Model.* **Diego A. Pizzagalli.** 2014, Annu. Rev. Clin. Psychol.

46. *Ventral striatal dopamine synthesis capacity is associated with individual differences in behavioral disinhibition.* **Andrew D. Lawrence, et.al.** March 2014, Frontiers in BEHAVIORAL NEUROSCIENCE.